THE JOY
OF LISTENING

an auditory training program

by

JANICE BALIKER LIGHT

Library of Congress Catalogue Card Number 78-52752

ISBN 0-88200-119-1

TABLE OF CONTENTS

Dedicated to my father, Tom.

INTRODUCTION

This is a program of auditory training consisting of 9 sections. It was designed for hearing-impaired students, but it can and has been used with children with learning disabilities who have weaknesses in the auditory areas.

The purpose of this program is to perfect listening skills and to improve:

- auditory discrimination
- auditory memory
- auditory attention span
- auditory sequencing, etc.

Students on this program have improved the use of their residual hearing, sharpened their listening skills, and have shown a general improvement in all auditory areas; they acquire a unique discipline for listening. Students have also shown improvement in reading and phonics.

Although auditory training is the primary purpose of this program, it is indeed possible and advisable to use many of these sections for teaching lipreading skills to hearing-impaired students.

GENERAL DIRECTIONS

When administering these lessons, the teacher should be seated at least 8-10 feet directly behind the student; no visual cues are used in listening exercises. Distance should depend upon the severity of the student's hearing impairment. If the student wears a hearing aid, it should be on the setting at which he usually wears it. These lessons can be administered in quiet or with background noise or music.

The teacher should have a copy of the lesson he is using with the student with the appropriate answers on it (circles, numbers, letters). In all sections the teacher fills in his own answers except section 5 for which answers are supplied. In Sections 1, 3, 4, and 5 the parentheses beside the titles on each page indicate what the student will be discriminating. These 9 sections do not have to be used in order, although some sections will be more difficult for some students than others.

These lessons can be used on a 1 to 1 basis or with small groups. The teacher says each item only once—never repeat an item. In all sections after the student has written a response he should indicate he is ready to listen to the next item by saying, "OK." This method has been found to be the most efficient and successful. If the student is not sure of the answer he should go on to the next item or write what he thought he heard. Before beginning any lesson the teacher should give clear directions to the student, perhaps a few practice items.

Each sheet is scored on a percentage basis. The score sheet will make each student's score meaningful, thus providing immediate reinforcement.

SCORE SHEET

100

90   Excellent
──
80   Very Good
──
70   Good
──
60

50   Fair, O.K.
──
40

30   Poor

20

10

0

SECTION I: CIRCLE THE WORD

Directions: Student reads orally the entire page to assure correct pronunciation. Teacher says, "Circle the word _____." The student
circles the word he heard. Then proceed to next set of words.

Example: Answer:

    miss   (miss)
    mice   mice

Teacher says, "Circle the word MISS." Student circles the word he
heard.

1

CIRCLE THE WORD (VOWEL SOUNDS)

| mitt | Mack | stack | peck |
| might | make | stake | peek |

| lit | lick | Dick | sack |
| light | like | dike | sake |

| sit | pick | den | rod |
| sight | pike | dean | rode |

| fit | tip | Ben | quack |
| fight | type | bean | quake |

| knit | rot | duck | will |
| night | wrote | duke | while |

| back | cot | cut | mill |
| bake | coat | cute | mile |

| rack | rat | miss | luck |
| rake | rate | mice | Luke |

| lack | at | tack | sin |
| lake | ate | take | sign |

| pill |
| pile |

CIRCLE THE WORD (VOWEL SOUNDS)

pin	fin	pet	tap
pine	fine	Pete	tape
dim	not	bed	cap
dime	note	bead	cape
hat	bit	ran	rip
hate	bite	rain	ripe
can	kit	men	Sam
cane	kite	mean	same
tin	set	ten	quit
tine	seat	teen	quite
tam	bet	met	whip
tame	beet	meat	wipe
win	net	mad	pad
wine	neat	made	paid
mat	wit	lad	red
mate	white	laid	read

Tim
time

33 items

CIRCLE THE WORD (VOWEL SOUNDS)

sock	fat	wet	mud
soak	fate	wheat	mood
rot	nap	fill	pass
wrote	nape	file	pace
bought	dead	kit	man
boat	deed	kite	mane
caught	fed	hit	tub
coat	feed	height	tube
cost	head	well	can
coast	heed	wheel	cane
con	led	set	nun
cone	lead	seat	noon
bass	bled	mass	pan
base	bleed	mace	pain
wed	said	lass	lamb
weed	seed	lace	lame
			dam
			dame

33 items

CIRCLE THE WORD (SHORT VOWELS)

mat	sun	pat	sad
met	sin	pet	sod
miss	ran	tin	cod
mess	run	tan	cud
man	sip	bag	fad
men	sap	beg	fed
cub	cap	big	fat
cob	cup	bug	fit
cot	red	bat	fan
cut	rod	but	fun
sat	dog	bit	rag
set	dug	bet	rug
dim	fig	tub	fog
dam	fog	tab	fig
rat	not	can	lid
rot	nut	con	led
			lass
			less

33 items

CIRCLE THE WORD (INITIAL BLENDS)

frail	trip	try	droop
trail	strip	cry	group
street	plaid	flew	scare
treat	glad	clue	spare
grain	glow	sting	pleat
brain	flow	string	fleet
bread	slow	breed	shy
dread	flow	greed	spy
cried	swim	smell	scream
tried	skim	spell	stream
sled	creek	brown	cream
fled	Greek	drown	dream
them	scared	shread	snare
stem	shared	spread	swear
tray	bride	speak	three
gray	dried	sneak	tree
			true
			crew

33 items

SECTION 2: WORD GROUPS

<u>Directions</u>: The student reads orally the first word group. The teacher says, "Number 1 is (word group)." The student writes a number 1 by the item he heard. The teacher says, "Number 2 is _____ _____." Student writes number 2 by the item he heard. Proceed in this manner for all 5 items in the group. Mix up the numbers for each item in each group.

<u>Example</u>:

____pine tree
____vine tree
____fine tea
____fine tree
____pine tea

<u>Answer</u>:

__3__pine tree
__1__vine tree
__2__fine tea
__4__fine tree
__5__pine tea

The teacher says, "Number 1 is VINE TREE." The student writes a number 1 in the blank next to the item he heard. The teacher says, "Number 2 is FINE TEA." The student writes a number 2 in the blank next to the item he heard. Proceed in this manner for all 5 items.

WORD GROUPS

____pine tree	____milk man	____cherry tart
____vine tree	____milk can	____cherry heart
____fine tea	____milk pan	____merry heart
____fine tree	____hill man	____cherry mart
____pine tea	____hill tan	____cherry dart
____rose hip	____spice cake	____ice skate
____rose whip	____iced cake	____nice wait
____nose whip	____rice cake	____ice lake
____toes hip	____nice steak	____nice lake
____rose lip	____nice cake	____rice lake
____milk shake	____red light	____fire place
____silk rake	____red night	____tire place
____milk cake	____red kite	____tire case
____silk cake	____head light	____fire race
____silk shake	____dead night	____fire plate
____good leader	____grape fruit	____bed room
____wood leader	____ape fruit	____red room
____good feeder	____ape suit	____bed broom
____good heater	____grape suit	____red broom
____wood heater	____cape fruit	____wed room
____bean soup	____in door	____tea time
____pea soup	____win more	____sea time
____green soup	____tin door	____tea lime
____green hoop	____win four	____sea lime
____bean loop	____win war	____tree lime
____hop scotch	____sweet potato	____day light
____stop watch	____sweet tomato	____bay light
____shop scotch	____eat potato	____day flight
____hot watch	____eat tomato	____bay flight
____hot scotch	____beat potato	____gay light
____kitty cat	____high roads	
____witty cat	____high toads	
____witty rat	____my roads	
____kitty mat	____my toads	
____kitty hat	____my goads	

100 items

WORD GROUPS

____two ways	____green eyes	____red rugs
____new ways	____cream pies	____red bugs
____who pays	____green ties	____bed bugs
____who stays	____green flies	____dead bugs
____two bays	____bean pies	____red mugs
____four cats	____tall owls	____same time
____more hats	____wall towels	____same dime
____poor cats	____small cows	____save mine
____four hats	____small towels	____save time
____sore cats	____hall towels	____save nine
____nine balls	____three bears	____this car
____nine dolls	____three chairs	____this far
____fine dolls	____free bears	____his car
____wine balls	____three hairs	____this star
____nine walls	____three mares	____his scar
____sad dogs	____fat boy	____right place
____mad dogs	____that boy	____night race
____glad dogs	____that toy	____white lace
____bad dogs	____bat boy	____light case
____sad hogs	____fat toy	____light taste
____white bees	____sweet ham	____many ways
____white cheese	____sweet jam	____many rays
____white keys	____neat tam	____any place
____light cheese	____sweet clam	____Penny plays
____light bees	____eat lamb	____Penny stays
____old men	____high time	____mad rat
____gold pen	____my dime	____sad cat
____gold hen	____my lime	____bad rat
____old hen	____dry lime	____sad hat
____cold men	____high crime	____bad bat
____red rose	____clear day	
____red nose	____dear May	
____red clothes	____near day	
____dead rose	____near bay	
____dead crows	____clear May	

100 items

WORD GROUPS

____dead goat	____lime pies	____brown cow
____red boat	____kind eyes	____brown towel
____fed goat	____fine skies	____brown fowl
____red note	____dime ties	____town towel
____red moat	____lime eyes	____town cow
____my mill	____that bear	____new books
____my will	____flat pear	____new cooks
____high hill	____that chair	____stew cooks
____dry hill	____fat mare	____two books
____my pill	____fat bear	____two cooks
____big lake	____pot hole	____fried eggs
____big cake	____hot roll	____dried eggs
____fig cake	____hot coal	____tried eggs
____pig bake	____hot pole	____dried kegs
____big rake	____shot mole	____tried kegs
____each week	____fair mate	____tight ring
____reach peak	____fair date	____white ring
____each beak	____rare date	____tight wing
____teach Greek	____rare mate	____white wing
____each peach	____fair bait	____light ring
____long wait	____mad man	____sun lamp
____wrong date	____sad man	____fun lamp
____long gate	____bad man	____sun camp
____wrong plate	____mad lamb	____fun camp
____long date	____sad lamb	____one lamp
____past hour	____seven hens	____sun roof
____last tower	____seven tens	____sun boot
____mass power	____seven pens	____fun boot
____last flower	____heaven scent	____fun roof
____fast shower	____heaven hens	____sun root
____two minks	____blue boys	
____few sinks	____blue toys	
____new drinks	____new toys	
____two drinks	____new boys	
____few minks	____two boys	

100 items

WORD GROUPS

____brown rice	____mail box	____sidewalk
____town rice	____mail blocks	____wide walk
____town price	____nail box	____tide walk
____brown price	____whale box	____wide rock
____crown price	____mail locks	____tide rock
____gold chain	____sweet coffee	____doormat
____gold cane	____sweet toffee	____more fat
____cold cane	____sweet taffy	____door cat
____cold chain	____wheat taffy	____poor cat
____cold pane	____wheat toffee	____sore cat
____ski slope	____someday	____inkwell
____ski soap	____Sunday	____pink well
____ski coat	____one day	____pink bell
____key coat	____Monday	____pink shell
____key slope	____fun day	____ink bell
____grape juice	____highway	____airplane
____grape goose	____sideway	____air lane
____grape moose	____Friday	____air pain
____drake juice	____high pay	____care plane
____straight juice	____fly bay	____pear plane
____old witch	____moon light	____baseball
____cold witch	____noon light	____lace doll
____old switch	____moon flight	____lace wall
____old twitch	____noon fight	____base doll
____cold switch	____spoon fight	____lace ball
____new glue	____housecoat	____oatmeal
____blue glue	____houseboat	____coat meal
____new clue	____house goat	____goat meal
____blue blue	____mouse coat	____goat peel
____blue clue	____mouse boat	____coat peel
____scare crow	____pan cake	
____scare show	____man lake	
____bear show	____bran cake	
____rare crow	____can cake	
____rare show	____bran flake	

100 items

SECTION 3: INDIVIDUAL WORDS

Directions: The student reads orally the first group of words. The teacher says, "Number 1 is (a word)." The student writes a number 1 by the word he heard. The teacher says, "Number 2 is _____." Student writes a number 2 by the word he heard. Proceed in this manner for all 5 words in the group. Mix up the numbers for each item in each group.

Example: Answer:

    _____cow   _3__ cow
    _____towel   _4__ towel
    _____chow   _2__ chow
    _____pow   _1__ pow
    _____growl   _5__ growl

    The teacher says, "Number 1 is POW." Student writes a number 1 in the blank next to the item he heard. Teacher says, "Number 2 is CHOW." Student writes a number 2 in the blank next to the item he heard. Proceed in this manner for all 5 items.

    Some of the words are repeated on the sheets to provide additional practice and repetition, which is extremely important in order to produce "disciplined listeners."

INDIVIDUAL WORDS (INITIAL CONSONANTS)

____bay	____cat	____gum	____men
____day	____hat	____hum	____den
____gay	____sat	____come	____hen
____hay	____fat	____some	____pen
____way	____bat	____rum	____ten

____see	____bug	____dot	____hop
____me	____rug	____got	____mop
____we	____hug	____hot	____pop
____bee	____dug	____lot	____top
____fee	____jug	____not	____shop

____pie	____mill	____can	____sad
____tie	____hill	____ran	____bad
____die	____will	____fan	____had
____lie	____kill	____man	____mad
____my	____fill	____pan	____dad

____no	____met	____pin	____name
____go	____bet	____win	____came
____hoe	____get	____fin	____game
____low	____let	____chin	____same
____toe	____net	____tin	____fame

____two	____sit	____bun	____call
____do	____fit	____fun	____hall
____who	____hit	____gun	____tall
____new	____it	____nun	____ball
____you	____bit	____sun	____fall

100 items

INDIVIDUAL WORDS (INITIAL CONSONANTS)

____had	____hat	____can	____ham
____mad	____sat	____man	____dam
____sad	____fat	____fan	____jam
____bad	____mat	____pan	____lamb
____dad	____bat	____ran	____tam

____pet	____pen	____red	____bell
____set	____hen	____bed	____well
____met	____men	____fed	____sell
____net	____ten	____Ted	____tell
____wet	____Ben	____wed	____fell

____pin	____fit	____dip	____mill
____tin	____sit	____hip	____kill
____win	____hit	____lip	____hill
____sin	____lit	____rip	____pill
____bin	____pit	____tip	____will

____not	____hop	____fog	____rock
____hot	____top	____dog	____dock
____pot	____mop	____hog	____lock
____dot	____pop	____log	____mock
____got	____cop	____bog	____sock

____bun	____bug	____but	____gum
____sun	____rug	____nut	____hum
____fun	____hug	____cut	____bum
____gun	____mug	____hut	____come
____run	____tug	____gut	____mum

100 items

16

INDIVIDUAL WORDS (INITIAL CONSONANTS)

____cow	____boy	____sit	____star
____vow	____toy	____lit	____far
____chow	____Roy	____bit	____car
____pow	____joy	____kit	____jar
____how	____coy	____fit	____tar
____bell	____time	____bat	____dear
____sell	____dime	____sat	____near
____tell	____rhyme	____cat	____cheer
____fell	____lime	____fat	____fear
____shell	____chime	____hat	____year
____see	____rose	____hot	____bear
____key	____toes	____caught	____care
____bee	____sews	____dot	____hair
____three	____those	____not	____chair
____she	____grows	____fought	____there
____beam	____hay	____but	____shoot
____dream	____say	____cut	____boot
____team	____gay	____nut	____root
____seem	____ray	____hut	____toot
____cream	____way	____shut	____suit
____mine	____two	____book	____cry
____line	____do	____cook	____try
____fine	____new	____look	____dry
____pine	____shoe	____took	____my
____shrine	____chew	____shook	____tie

100 items

INDIVIDUAL WORDS (INITIAL CONSONANTS)

____sort	____last	____sand	____card
____fort	____mast	____band	____hard
____port	____vast	____hand	____lard
____court	____fast	____land	____bard
____sport	____past	____stand	____yard
____miss	____cold	____dark	____cash
____kiss	____fold	____bark	____sash
____this	____hold	____park	____mash
____hiss	____sold	____hark	____rash
____sis	____told	____mark	____dash
____wink	____itch	____arm	____peach
____link	____pitch	____farm	____teach
____mink	____ditch	____harm	____beach
____pink	____witch	____charm	____reach
____sink	____hitch	____alarm	____leach
____heard	____sang	____camp	____cork
____bird	____tang	____lamp	____fork
____word	____fang	____ramp	____pork
____curd	____hang	____vamp	____stork
____gird	____pang	____stamp	____work
____catch	____sack	____dust	____waste
____patch	____back	____must	____haste
____hatch	____pack	____rust	____paste
____match	____quack	____gust	____taste
____batch	____tack	____bust	____baste

100 items

INDIVIDUAL WORDS (INITIAL CONSONANTS)

____hung	____song	____merge	____beast
____lung	____long	____dirge	____feast
____rung	____wrong	____purge	____least
____sung	____tong	____serge	____yeast
____stung	____bong	____urge	____priest
____hutch	____barge	____belt	____burn
____such	____large	____melt	____churn
____touch	____sarge	____felt	____turn
____much	____charge	____welt	____fern
____dutch	____Marge	____knelt	____learn
____neck	____catch	____sound	____prince
____peck	____match	____bound	____mince
____deck	____patch	____found	____rinse
____check	____hatch	____hound	____since
____wreck	____latch	____mound	____wince
____dirt	____hush	____built	____sunk
____hurt	____mush	____tilt	____chunk
____pert	____rush	____wilt	____bunk
____skirt	____gush	____guilt	____hunk
____shirt	____lush	____quilt	____punk
____lunch	____worst	____roast	____birch
____punch	____burst	____boast	____church
____bunch	____first	____host	____perch
____hunch	____cursed	____most	____search
____munch	____thirst	____post	____lurch

100 items

INDIVIDUAL WORDS (INITIAL CONSONANTS)

____back	____boot	____more	____size
____pack	____toot	____poor	____wise
____shack	____root	____your	____pies
____tack	____loot	____door	____ties
____rack	____suit	____four	____rise
____sick	____vase	____mail	____toes
____lick	____face	____tail	____goes
____pick	____base	____jail	____sews
____quick	____race	____nail	____shows
____wick	____lace	____pail	____throws
____light	____sink	____sell	____ax
____right	____wink	____tell	____tax
____fight	____think	____bell	____Max
____white	____pink	____well	____jacks
____night	____mink	____yell	____quacks
____test	____back	____bun	____map
____best	____pack	____sun	____nap
____nest	____sack	____gun	____cap
____west	____quack	____run	____lap
____rest	____Jack	____done	____rap
____whip	____stop	____hold	____an
____ship	____hop	____gold	____can
____sip	____shop	____told	____tan
____dip	____pop	____sold	____ran
____rip	____drop	____mold	____man

100 items

20

INDIVIDUAL WORDS (INITIAL CONSONANTS)

____sick	____belt	____kind	____kill
____pick	____melt	____find	____fill
____kick	____welt	____wind	____hill
____lick	____felt	____mind	____pill
____thick	____dealt	____hind	____will

____fast	____test	____pearl	____bent
____past	____pest	____curl	____rent
____cast	____nest	____girl	____dent
____last	____rest	____hurl	____went
____mast	____vest	____swirl	____vent

____wing	____guest	____born	____salt
____sing	____west	____corn	____malt
____king	____zest	____horn	____vault
____thing	____best	____torn	____halt
____ring	____quest	____worn	____fault

____bell	____boast	____call	____rock
____sell	____ghost	____hall	____gawk
____tell	____most	____tall	____walk
____well	____post	____wall	____dock
____fell	____roast	____ball	____lock

____bath	____tint	____tart	____mock
____math	____hint	____cart	____sock
____path	____lint	____heart	____shock
____hath	____mint	____part	____chalk
____rath	____dint	____mart	____knock

100 items

INDIVIDUAL WORDS (INITIAL CONSONANTS & BLENDS)

____moose	____born	____car	____roll
____goose	____horn	____tar	____hole
____use	____corn	____far	____bowl
____juice	____worn	____star	____mole
____loose	____morn	____scar	____pole
____should	____or	____came	____seal
____good	____nor	____game	____feel
____wood	____door	____same	____heel
____stood	____more	____name	____wheel
____hood	____poor	____lame	____meal
____moon	____ox	____part	____blow
____noon	____box	____dart	____snow
____soon	____fox	____art	____know
____spoon	____rocks	____heart	____crow
____tune	____socks	____mart	____grow
____cool	____clock	____nose	____brown
____wool	____rock	____rose	____town
____full	____sock	____goes	____clown
____pull	____block	____hose	____crown
____tool	____knock	____pose	____down
____book	____caught	____ride	____boat
____cook	____taught	____hide	____coat
____took	____thought	____side	____wrote
____look	____brought	____tide	____dote
____shook	____bought	____wide	____goat

100 items

INDIVIDUAL WORDS (INITIAL CONSONANTS & BLENDS)

____rock	____gem	____vine	____flew
____clock	____them	____shine	____clue
____shock	____stem	____wine	____dew
____smock	____hem	____spine	____stew
____block	____flem	____line	____blew
____tack	____chin	____pray	____yell
____crack	____win	____gray	____bell
____shack	____pin	____way	____well
____pack	____grin	____they	____fell
____track	____thin	____stay	____shell
____neck	____swim	____rich	____sit
____check	____dim	____switch	____quit
____peck	____brim	____pitch	____wit
____wreck	____grim	____ditch	____lit
____speck	____slim	____stitch	____knit
____stick	____mass	____train	____jump
____chick	____crass	____rain	____stump
____wick	____class	____lain	____lump
____brick	____gas	____slain	____bump
____pick	____grass	____brain	____grump
____clam	____drill	____wheel	____shook
____yam	____spill	____veal	____book
____jam	____kill	____meal	____look
____gram	____will	____seal	____cook
____sham	____fill	____kneel	____rook

100 items

INDIVIDUAL WORDS (INITIAL CONSONANTS & BLENDS)

____horn	____cash	____rush	____round
____corn	____mash	____hush	____found
____born	____rash	____mush	____hound
____torn	____dash	____gush	____pound
____morn	____lash	____thrush	____sound
____dark	____most	____match	____shirt
____bark	____toast	____patch	____dirt
____park	____roast	____hatch	____hurt
____mark	____ghost	____batch	____skirt
____hark	____host	____catch	____pert
____raise	____paste	____bump	____bird
____haze	____taste	____dump	____word
____ways	____waste	____hump	____heard
____gaze	____baste	____jump	____third
____graze	____haste	____lump	____purred
____find	____beach	____lamp	____mile
____mind	____peach	____camp	____smile
____rind	____reach	____damp	____file
____kind	____teach	____ramp	____while
____hind	____bleach	____stamp	____pile
____ten	____best	____curl	____ought
____men	____nest	____girl	____thought
____hen	____test	____hurl	____caught
____den	____rest	____pearl	____bought
____pen	____pest	____whirl	____sought

100 items

INDIVIDUAL WORDS (INITIAL CONSONANTS & BLENDS)

____bat	____come	____shine	____oil
____fat	____some	____pine	____boil
____sat	____chum	____wine	____foil
____chat	____plum	____fine	____soil
____flat	____thumb	____line	____toil
____pen	____bout	____wink	____where
____when	____out	____pink	____share
____ten	____pout	____sink	____pear
____hen	____gout	____link	____fare
____glen	____doubt	____think	____lair
____ship	____shoot	____me	____power
____trip	____suit	____we	____flower
____dip	____cute	____she	____shower
____flip	____boot	____fee	____tower
____lip	____loot	____key	____sour
____chop	____book	____shake	____car
____mop	____took	____make	____bar
____hop	____shook	____wake	____far
____drop	____hook	____cake	____jar
____stop	____brook	____lake	____star
____fire	____more	____whirl	____gem
____wire	____four	____pearl	____them
____tire	____door	____curl	____hem
____shire	____core	____swirl	____stem
____hire	____floor	____girl	____flem

100 items

INDIVIDUAL WORDS (INITIAL CONSONANTS & BLENDS)

____flag	____rock	____boat	____gold
____bag	____clock	____goat	____cold
____rag	____lock	____coat	____fold
____brag	____mock	____float	____hold
____lag	____sock	____gloat	____sold
____buck	____will	____mash	____moss
____luck	____kill	____cash	____loss
____truck	____dill	____dash	____cross
____suck	____fill	____lash	____boss
____stuck	____chill	____flash	____toss
____back	____rain	____hush	____ship
____sack	____chain	____mush	____chip
____shack	____main	____flush	____flip
____lack	____pain	____blush	____hip
____stack	____brain	____crush	____sip
____peck	____paid	____day	____pan
____deck	____maid	____pay	____can
____check	____laid	____pray	____man
____neck	____raid	____say	____ran
____wreck	____braid	____may	____tan
____sick	____nail	____clay	____peg
____chick	____pail	____gay	____leg
____pick	____fail	____hay	____beg
____tick	____mail	____lay	____egg
____wick	____rail	____ray	____keg

100 items

INDIVIDUAL WORDS (INITIAL VOICED CONSONANTS)

____day	____bet	____late	____bear
____bay	____get	____mate	____rare
____way	____wet	____date	____wear
____gay	____let	____wait	____dare
____may	____met	____rate	____mare
____me	____mat	____zone	____man
____we	____rat	____bone	____van
____be	____bat	____lone	____ran
____lee	____gnat	____roan	____ban
____knee	____vat	____moan	____Dan
____buy	____mitt	____night	____mill
____my	____lit	____right	____dill
____lie	____bit	____light	____gill
____die	____wit	____mite	____will
____guy	____knit	____bite	____Jill
____go	____but	____boat	____lash
____no	____nut	____goat	____mash
____low	____gut	____note	____rash
____row	____rut	____wrote	____dash
____Joe	____mutt	____vote	____bash
____do	____dot	____moon	____doze
____zoo	____not	____noon	____goes
____moo	____lot	____room	____mows
____new	____got	____doom	____nose
____boo	____rot	____boom	____rose

100 items

INDIVIDUAL WORDS (INITIAL UNVOICED CONSONANTS)

____pay	____cat	____shed	____tin
____say	____fat	____fed	____chin
____hay	____pat	____Ted	____sin
____Kay	____chat	____head	____fin
____Fay	____hat	____said	____pin

____pie	____sit	____sort	____sheep
____hi	____fit	____port	____cheap
____shy	____hit	____fort	____keep
____tie	____pit	____short	____heap
____why	____kit	____court	____seep

____he	____hot	____pad	____chop
____she	____cot	____sad	____top
____tea	____tot	____fad	____hop
____key	____fought	____had	____pop
____see	____pot	____shad	____shop

____toe	____shut	____her	____keys
____so	____hut	____purr	____tease
____show	____cut	____sir	____cheese
____hoe	____what	____cur	____she's
____foe	____putt	____fir	____he's

____sue	____chow	____kite	____hose
____chew	____towel	____tight	____pose
____two	____foul	____fight	____sews
____who	____cow	____sight	____toes
____shoe	____how	____white	____chose

100 items

INDIVIDUAL WORDS (INITIAL BLENDS)

____pray	____chow	____shed	____gray
____stay	____growl	____sled	____spray
____play	____plow	____spread	____tray
____clay	____thou	__ _bread	____they
____they	____brow	____fled	____stray

____tree	____shot	____slow	____thrill
____three	____thought	____glow	____still
____she	____brought	____blow	____spill
____flee	____trot	____though	____quill
____glee	____spot	____flow	____chill

____spy	____spin	____breeze	____fry
____try	____thin	____please	____try
____cry	____chin	____freeze	____shy
____dry	____skin	____cheese	____spry
____sky	____grin	____these	____sty

____flow	____swum	____blue	____chick
____throw	____from	____glue	____quick
____slow	____drum	____chew	____trick
____blow	____thumb	____through	____stick
____grow	____crumb	____flew	____thick

____clue	____snap	____shake	____trip
____flew	____trap	____flake	____ship
____stew	____flap	____break	____chip
____shoe	____clap	____steak	____flip
____true	____slap	____snake	____clip

100 items

INDIVIDUAL WORDS (MEDIAL CONSONANTS)

____camel	____bubble	____fatten	____waiter
____castle	____bundle	____fashion	____wafer
____candle	____buckle	____faction	____waster
____cattle	____bustle	____fasten	____wager
____cackle	____bumble	____famine	____waver

____butter	____sipper	____money	____armor
____buzzer	____sitter	____muddy	____archer
____buffer	____simmer	____mummy	____arbor
____bumper	____sister	____mushy	____ardor
____buster	____sifter	____musty	____author

____paper	____cover	____later	____liver
____pacer	____cutter	____labor	____lifter
____pastor	____color	____layer	____litter
____painter	____Custer	____lamer	____lisper
____paver	____comer	____laser	____licker

____father	____azure	____wisher	____leader
____farther	____actor	____winter	____leaner
____foster	____answer	____winner	____leaper
____farmer	____after	____whisper	____liter
____fonder	____anger	____wither	____leisure

____letter	____bother	____matter	____ladder
____lever	____boxer	____manner	____lather
____leather	____bomber	____master	____lancer
____leper	____barber	____madder	____laughter
____lesser	____bopper	____masher	____lacquer

100 items

INDIVIDUAL WORDS (FINAL CONSONANTS)

____ape	____end	____pan	____wig
____ache	____edge	____pass	____win
____ace	____ebb	____path	____whip
____aim	____etch	____patch	____which
____aid	____egg	____pack	____wish
____eve	____add	____need	____rag
____each	____am	____niece	____rash
____eat	____an	____knees	____ranch
____eel	____ash	____near	____rat
____ease	____at	____neat	____rats
____I'd	____on	____road	____bone
____ice	____all	____robe	____both
____eyes	____off	____wrote	____boat
____I'm	____odd	____rose	____boast
____I've	____ox	____rope	____bowl
____own	____hut	____sash	____cat
____oaf	____hush	____sack	____cash
____ode	____hum	____Sam	____cab
____oat	____hug	____sand	____can
____oats	____hub	____sad	____cats
____if	____bat	____pig	____came
____it	____ban	____pit	____cage
____in	____band	____pick	____cane
____itch	____bad	____pitch	____case
____ink	____batch	____pink	____cave

100 items

INDIVIDUAL WORDS (FINAL CONSONANTS)

____cheese	____place	____stag	____trash
____cheat	____plate	____stab	____trap
____cheap	____plan	____stand	____track
____chief	____plays	____stack	____tramp
____cheek	____plague	____stash	____tracked
____shade	____grade	____grove	____trace
____shame	____graze	____growth	____train
____shave	____grape	____groan	____trade
____shape	____grace	____gross	____trait
____share	____grate	____grows	____traced
____slip	____slime	____creek	____grease
____slick	____slice	____creep	____greet
____slim	____slight	____crease	____green
____slit	____slide	____creed	____greed
____slid	____slides	____cream	____grief
____brave	____strike	____stuck	____skim
____brace	____strive	____stung	____skin
____brain	____stripe	____stuff	____skid
____braid	____strife	____stub	____skip
____break	____stride	____stunt	____skit
____bran	____fret	____state	____crack
____brag	____fresh	____stage	____crash
____brass	____Fred	____stale	____crab
____brad	____friend	____stain	____cram
____brash	____frets	____stave	____crass

100 items

INDIVIDUAL WORDS (FINAL CONSONANTS)

____age	____ham	____seen	____map
____ape	____hat	____seed	____mat
____ate	____had	____seem	____mad
____ace	____has	____seat	____man
____aim	____have	____seal	____mass
____ease	____bed	____live	____less
____each	____bell	____lid	____led
____eve	____bet	____lip	____leg
____east	____best	____lit	____left
____eel	____beg	____list	____lend
____eye	____lime	____cane	____rob
____ice	____line	____cake	____rod
____eyes	____like	____came	____rot
____I'm	____life	____cage	____rock
____I've	____light	____cape	____ross
____own	____lake	____game	____white
____owes	____lame	____gate	____wise
____ore	____lane	____gave	____wide
____ode	____lace	____gain	____wine
____oats	____late	____gaze	____wipe
____pet	____cap	____fan	____wheat
____pen	____cat	____fat	____weep
____pep	____can	____fast	____weed
____peck	____cab	____fad	____week
____peg	____cash	____fact	____weave

100 items

INDIVIDUAL WORDS (FINAL CONSONANTS & BLENDS)

____art	____harsh	____past	____dent
____ark	____harp	____patch	____desk
____arch	____heart	____pact	____death
____arm	____hark	____path	____deck
____arched	____harm	____patched	____dense
____mast	____cord	____bard	____tend
____mask	____corn	____bark	____tent
____match	____cork	____barn	____tense
____mash	____court	____barge	____tenth
____matched	____corpse	____barbed	____test
____mark	____cash	____fork	____curd
____mart	____catch	____form	____curl
____marsh	____cast	____fort	____curt
____march	____cask	____fourth	____curb
____Mars	____can't	____forced	____kirsch
____with	____last	____ramp	____rift
____wish	____lash	____ranch	____ridge
____wisk	____latch	____rash	____wrist
____witch	____lass	____rant	____risk
____wince	____laughed	____rank	____rinse
____birth	____part	____list	____hurt
____birch	____park	____lick	____herd
____bird	____parse	____lisp	____herb
____burn	____parch	____lift	____hearse
____burst	____parked	____limp	____hers

100 items

INDIVIDUAL WORDS (FINAL VOICED CONSONANTS)

____has	____lean	____bade	____game
____have	____leaves	____babe	____gain
____had	____lead	____bathe	____gaze
____ham	____leave	____bays	____gave
____hand	____league	____beige	____gauge
____cage	____lodge	____rise	____fame
____cane	____lawn	____ride	____fain
____came	____long	____rhyme	____fade
____cave	____log	____rind	____phase
____kale	____laud	____writhe	____fades
____rove	____cob	____tab	____fag
____roam	____cod	____tag	____fad
____rose	____calm	____tam	____fan
____robe	____cause	____tan	____fang
____rode	____con	____tad	____fans
____rage	____rid	____pain	____done
____raise	____rib	____page	____does
____raid	____rig	____pave	____dumb
____rain	____rim	____paid	____dug
____rave	____ridge	____pays	____dove
____lays	____loan	____sad	____dime
____laid	____load	____sag	____dine
____lame	____lobe	____sand	____dies
____lane	____loam	____Sam	____dive
____lathe	____loathe	____salve	____died

100 items

INDIVIDUAL WORDS (FINAL UNVOICED CONSONANTS)

____mat	____cop	____peep	____reap
____map	____cost	____peace	____reef
____mash	____cot	____peak	____reach
____mass	____cough	____peach	____wreath
____match	____coughed	____Pete	____reek
____pat	____wit	____cat	____hat
____pass	____wish	____cap	____half
____pack	____witch	____calf	____hash
____path	____whip	____catch	____hatch
____patch	____with	____cash	____hast
____cat	____sis	____rat	____dip
____cap	____sit	____rack	____ditch
____cash	____sip	____raft	____dish
____catch	____sift	____rash	____dips
____cast	____sick	____wrap	____Dick
____last	____lip	____beef	____pep
____lap	____lick	____beet	____pet
____lash	____list	____beach	____peck
____lass	____lit	____beep	____pest
____laugh	____lisp	____beast	____pets
____bat	____rich	____leak	____desk
____back	____rip	____leap	____debt
____bass	____rift	____leach	____deaf
____batch	____wrist	____lease	____death
____bath	____Rick	____least	____deck

100 items

INDIVIDUAL WORDS (R VARIATIONS)

____far	____purr	____door	____stare
____for	____par	____dire	____steer
____fur	____pier	____dare	____store
____fear	____poor	____dear	____star
____fire	____pure	____doer	____stir

____wire	____tar	____lair	____spare
____where	____tear	____leer	____spear
____wore	____tier	____liar	____spore
____were	____tore	____lore	____spire
____we're	____tire	____lure	____spur

____car	____sore	____are	____sneer
____core	____sure	____ear	____snore
____cure	____sir	____or	____snare
____care	____sour	____air	____smear
____cur	____seer	____our	____smart

____bar	____sheer	____hair	____bairn
____bear	____shore	____here	____baron
____bore	____share	____hire	____born
____beer	____shire	____her	____barn
____burr	____shower	____hour	____burn

____mar	____cheer	____scare	____curd
____mere	____chair	____scour	____card
____mare	____char	____scar	____cord
____more	____chore	____score	____cared
____myrrh	____churr	____skier	____cured

100 items

INDIVIDUAL WORDS (SHORT VOWELS)

____bat	____last	____sack	____track
____bet	____list	____sick	____trek
____bit	____lost	____sock	____trick
____bought	____lust	____suck	____rock
____but	____lest	____check	____truck

____pat	____lack	____bad	____bag
____pet	____lick	____bed	____beg
____pit	____lock	____bid	____big
____putt	____luck	____bud	____bog
____pot	____fleck	____mod	____bug

____kit	____bell	____lad	____well
____cat	____bill	____led	____will
____caught	____ball	____lid	____wall
____cut	____bowl	____laud	____wool
____get	____bull	____flood	____wow

____net	____pan	____sat	____bag
____knit	____pen	____set	____big
____not	____pin	____sit	____bog
____nut	____pawn	____sought	____bug
____gnat	____pun	____shut	____beg

____mass	____tan	____bass	____check
____mess	____ten	____Bess	____chick
____miss	____tin	____boss	____chalk
____moss	____ton	____bus	____chuck
____muss	____con	____bliss	____chap

100 items

INDIVIDUAL WORDS (LONG VOWELS)

_____bay	_____sane	_____share	_____lay
_____bee	_____seen	_____sheer	_____lee
_____buy	_____sign	_____shire	_____lie
_____bow	_____sewn	_____shore	_____low
_____boo	_____soon	_____sure	_____Lou

_____day	_____raid	_____fare	_____say
_____dee	_____reed	_____fear	_____see
_____die	_____ride	_____fire	_____sigh
_____dough	_____rode	_____for	_____so
_____do	_____rude	_____fur	_____sue

_____hay	_____pail	_____laid	_____mate
_____he	_____peel	_____lead	_____meet
_____high	_____pile	_____lied	_____might
_____ho	_____pole	_____load	_____moat
_____who	_____pull	_____lewd	_____mute

_____dame	_____mail	_____tame	_____tail
_____deem	_____meal	_____team	_____teal
_____dime	_____mile	_____time	_____tile
_____dome	_____mole	_____tome	_____toll
_____doom	_____mule	_____tomb	_____tool

_____bait	_____stale	_____rail	_____dale
_____beet	_____steel	_____reel	_____deal
_____bite	_____style	_____rile	_____dial
_____boat	_____stole	_____roll	_____dole
_____boot	_____stool	_____rule	_____duel

100 items

SECTION 4: ONE-TWO-THREE

Directions: The student reads orally the entire page to assure correct pronunciation of each word.

Starting with the first group of words, the teacher says 3 words "consecutively," in any order. The student puts a number 1 by the word he heard first, a number 2 by the word he heard next, and a number 3 by the word he heard last.

Example:

      ____tea
      ____me
      ____he

Answer:

      _3_ tea
      _1_ me
      _2_ he

Teacher says, "ME, HE, TEA." Student writes a number 1 in the blank next to ME, a number 2 by HE, and a number 3 by TEA.

1-2-3 (INITIAL CONSONANTS & BLENDS)

____fib	____rid	____dig	____trap
____rib	____kid	____pig	____cap
____bib	____lid	____jig	____lap
____near	____kiss	____pit	____cast
____fear	____miss	____fit	____last
____rear	____hiss	____wit	____fast
____bad	____calf	____rag	____beg
____fad	____laugh	____bag	____leg
____lad	____staff	____sag	____keg
____ball	____ram	____hand	____lip
____call	____lamb	____land	____hip
____fall	____dam	____band	____chip
____car	____star	____pass	____tab
____bar	____jar	____mass	____cab
____far	____far	____lass	____scab
____mat	____wreck	____wed	____bath
____rat	____deck	____head	____rath
____hat	____neck	____dead	____math
____bend	____hatch	____felt	____sap
____lend	____match	____belt	____map
____mend	____latch	____melt	____flap
____rim	____mix	____mash	____back
____dim	____fix	____rash	____black
____him	____six	____hash	____pack
____west			
____test			
____rest			

99 items

1-2-3 (INITIAL CONSONANTS & BLENDS)

____wade	____rave	____meal	____nail
____trade	____slave	____kneel	____pail
____grade	____save	____peel	____sail
____tape	____reach	____keen	____shave
____cape	____beach	____lean	____cave
____ape	____teach	____clean	____gave
____brave	____seal	____niece	____creed
____crave	____deal	____piece	____greed
____grave	____real	____geese	____read
____leaf	____seen	____lane	____seek
____beef	____bean	____cane	____peek
____thief	____dean	____vane	____weak
____feel	____crease	____dare	____deem
____wheel	____grease	____fair	____dream
____heel	____lease	____mare	____cream
____steam	____whale	____speed	____jeep
____ream	____pale	____bleed	____leap
____gleam	____scale	____need	____heep
____tease	____chair	____leak	____preach
____bees	____scare	____meek	____peach
____fees	____pair	____cheek	____bleach
____cage	____feed	____beam	____weep
____rage	____deed	____seam	____deep
____page	____weed	____team	____seep
____shape			
____drape			
____grape			

99 items

1-2-3 (INITIAL CONSONANTS & BLENDS)

____pear	____hem	____blond	____lawn
____scare	____gem	____frond	____fawn
____dare	____them	____bond	____pawn
____knob	____wax	____call	____cot
____cob	____lax	____tall	____got
____job	____tax	____mall	____dot
____off	____shock	____floss	____clock
____cough	____flock	____loss	____block
____scoff	____stock	____boss	____dock
____mess	____broth	____pot	____shop
____less	____cloth	____hot	____crop
____press	____moth	____plot	____drop
____rock	____hex	____rang	____fought
____sock	____sex	____hang	____caught
____mock	____vex	____bang	____thought
____hog	____stare	____wall	____ball
____log	____share	____crawl	____hall
____bog	____hare	____drawl	____fall
____bet	____song	____frost	____toss
____net	____long	____cost	____moss
____debt	____wrong	____lost	____cross
____rod	____held	____thing	____bought
____cod	____weld	____sing	____rot
____pod	____geld	____ring	____brought
____clog			
____dog			
____flog			

99 items

1-2-3 (INITIAL CONSONANTS & BLENDS)

____tub	____mug	____town	____cuff
____rub	____jug	____down	____rough
____cub	____lug	____clown	____fluff
____gruff	____drum	____skate	____gum
____muff	____come	____bait	____rum
____puff	____mum	____date	____hum
____fun	____must	____race	____round
____run	____dust	____trace	____found
____bun	____ trust	____base	____hound
____rust	____cloud	____bud	____cook
____bust	____loud	____mud	____took
____lust	____proud	____blood	____book
____spout	____maid	____king	____blouse
____gout	____laid	____sting	____mouse
____pout	____raid	____bring	____house
____mate	____lace	____damp	____shower
____fate	____face	____ramp	____tower
____date	____mace	____camp	____flower
____lame	____chuck	____best	____break
____tame	____truck	____guest	____flake
____name	____stuck	____jest	____shake
____buck	____rush	____hour	____chain
____duck	____hush	____sour	____train
____luck	____mush	____power	____brain
____bump			
____lump			
____dump			

99 items

44

1-2-3 (INITIAL CONSONANTS & BLENDS)

____knees	____trial	____tight	____rose
____trees	____tile	____trite	____froze
____freeze	____pile	____fright	____hose
____cried	____bind	____home	____hide
____fried	____mind	____dome	____side
____dried	____find	____comb	____ride
____while	____bright	____price	____mile
____dial	____right	____rice	____smile
____file	____sight	____vice	____tile
____line	____roast	____life	____swine
____fine	____boast	____wife	____wine
____sign	____toast	____knife	____vine
____height	____mice	____rhyme	____white
____light	____nice	____prime	____bite
____might	____lice	____grime	____fight
____goal	____guide	____wise	____ode
____coal	____wide	____rise	____rode
____bowl	____bride	____size	____load
____cope	____time	____hive	____loan
____hope	____dime	____five	____moan
____soap	____lime	____dive	____bone
____breeze	____ripe	____cone	____stove
____flees	____wipe	____phone	____cove
____keys	____type	____bone	____rove
____died			
____lied			
____slide			

99 items

1-2-3 (INITIAL CONSONANTS & BLENDS)

____should	____thick	____sty	____feed
____could	____stick	____shy	____seed
____stood	____sick	____thy	____she'd
____shoot	____fought	____shread	____cold
____cute	____shot	____thread	____fold
____suit	____thought	____Fred	____sold
____sheet	____fine	____sue	____crawl
____cheat	____shine	____shoe	____shawl
____feet	____thine	____chew	____brawl
____sheep	____chat	____ship	____chill
____cheap	____fat	____chip	____kill
____jeep	____that	____sip	____still
____seen	____sold	____shop	____fool
____sheen	____cold	____stop	____stool
____jean	____fold	____chop	____cool
____feel	____sew	____cap	____jaw
____seal	____Joe	____sap	____saw
____steal	____show	____chap	____thaw
____fell	____gin	____Jack	____chain
____shell	____thin	____stack	____Jane
____jell	____shin	____shack	____stain
____she	____stay	____shake	____chief
____fee	____say	____steak	____thief
____thee	____they	____cake	____sheaf
____stem			
____them			
____gem			

99 items

1-2-3 (INITIAL CONSONANTS & BLENDS)

____big	____fish	____key	____dip
____wig	____dish	____me	____rip
____fig	____wish	____he	____flip
____hug	____shoe	____hill	____met
____bug	____blue	____pill	____yet
____rug	____new	____will	____set
____top	____took	____that	____my
____mop	____book	____cat	____shy
____hop	____cook	____mat	____sky
____bed	____she	____had	____wet
____said	____he	____sad	____pet
____fed	____bee	____dad	____get
____but	____say	____two	____jam
____what	____pay	____who	____tam
____cut	____tray	____chew	____ham
____pie	____no	____boat	____chin
____tie	____row	____coat	____pin
____lie	____blow	____note	____thin
____men	____box	____pick	____cool
____hen	____fox	____sick	____wool
____pen	____lox	____lick	____fool
____fan	____twin	____how	____wire
____tan	____tin	____now	____tire
____pan	____spin	____chow	____fire
____yell			
____fell			
____tell			

99 items

1-2-3 (INITIAL BLENDS)

____clap	____tree	____flake	____grill
____slap	____free	____steak	____thrill
____flap	____spree	____shake	____drill
____try	____trim	____street	____cheek
____cry	____grim	____sheet	____sneak
____dry	____brim	____treat	____speak
____sky	____frown	____gram	____swell
____shy	____drown	____scram	____smell
____fry	____crown	____dram	____shell
____flow	____trick	____chum	____thread
____slow	____brick	____plum	____bread
____blow	____stick	____slum	____dread
____clue	____glad	____freeze	____brace
____flew	____plaid	____breeze	____trace
____glue	____clad	____trees	____grace
____spill	____trip	____smoke	____price
____chill	____grip	____spoke	____slice
____still	____drip	____broke	____thrice
____pray	____clip	____prone	____swim
____gray	____slip	____groan	____skim
____tray	____flip	____thrown	____slim
____slay	____train	____drew	____bloom
____play	____brain	____grew	____gloom
____clay	____strain	____threw	____plume
____fly			
____sly			
____shy			

99 items

48

1-2-3 (FINAL CONSONANTS)

____arm	____man	____rice	____fade
____art	____mad	____rhyme	____face
____arch	____map	____right	____fame
____bar	____mug	____raise	____feed
____bark	____muff	____raid	____feet
____barn	____much	____rage	____fees
____rip	____tub	____road	____lime
____rib	____tuck	____roam	____line
____rid	____tug	____rose	____like
____bat	____pan	____root	____leek
____bag	____pass	____room	____lease
____bass	____pat	____roof	____lead
____cab	____run	____mood	____meat
____can	____rug	____moon	____meek
____cat	____rub	____moose	____mean
____rag	____rot	____cake	____need
____rat	____rock	____case	____neat
____ram	____rob	____came	____niece
____six	____read	____bean	____peace
____sick	____reep	____beam	____peek
____sin	____reef	____bees	____peel
____seen	____save	____bake	____lace
____seed	____sane	____bait	____lame
____seat	____sake	____base	____lane
____lack			
____lad			
____lab			

99 items

1-2-3 (FINAL BLENDS)

____art	____hunch	____heart	____rank
____arm	____hunt	____harm	____ramp
____arch	____hung	____hard	____ranch
____mark	____church	____pork	____lark
____march	____chirp	____port	____lard
____mart	____churn	____porch	____large
____burn	____cart	____perk	____rinse
____bird	____card	____purge	____rink
____birth	____carp	____pearl	____ring
____word	____park	____sand	____ranch
____work	____parse	____sang	____rank
____worm	____parch	____sash	____rant
____darn	____hurt	____horse	____bent
____dark	____heard	____horn	____bend
____dart	____hurl	____horde	____bench
____curb	____ford	____starch	____wing
____curl	____form	____start	____wish
____curd	____fork	____starve	____wind
____corn	____dense	____storm	____wash
____cord	____dent	____stork	____wasp
____cork	____death	____stored	____want
____bark	____chart	____lift	____month
____barn	____charm	____lisp	____monk
____bard	____charge	____list	____mush
____ant			
____ask			
____ash			

99 items

50

1-2-3 (SHORT VOWELS)

____mass	____tell	____lass	____sing
____mess	____toll	____less	____sang
____miss	____till	____loss	____sung
____last	____let	____lock	____ring
____lost	____lot	____lick	____rang
____list	____lit	____luck	____rung
____nut	____mud	____deck	____shad
____net	____mad	____dock	____shed
____not	____mod	____duck	____shod
____top	____bat	____cab	____mash
____tip	____but	____cub	____mesh
____tap	____bit	____cob	____mush
____set	____pun	____sick	____spat
____sat	____pin	____sack	____spit
____sit	____pan	____sock	____spot
____tam	____ram	____tick	____stack
____Tom	____rim	____tack	____stick
____Tim	____rum	____tuck	____stock
____bend	____lag	____rat	____must
____band	____leg	____rut	____mast
____bond	____log	____rot	____mist
____pick	____lad	____rib	____track
____pack	____led	____rob	____trick
____peck	____lid	____rub	____truck
____hat			
____hot			
____hut			

99 items

SECTION 5: FILL IN THE BLANK

Directions: Teacher says the first word. According to what he heard, the student fills in the blank with the sound. Teacher proceeds to next word, etc. Teacher will have answers for this section.

Example: Answer:

       ____ob   j ob
       ____ob   c ob
       ____ob   r ob
       ____ob   s ob
       ____ob   m ob

     Teacher says, "JOB." Student writes a "j" in the first blank. Teacher says, "COB." Students writes a "c" in the second blank. Teacher says, "ROB." Student writes "r" in the third blank. Teacher says, "SOB." Student writes "s" in the fourth blank. Teacher says, "MOB." Student writes "m" in the next blank.

FILL IN THE BLANK (INITIAL CONSONANT)

_____oom	_____ake	_____ale	_____ave
_____oom	_____ake	_____ale	_____ave
_____oom	_____ake	___ __ale	_____ave
_____oom	_____ake	_____ale	_____ave
_____oom	_____ake	_____ale	_____ave

_____ool	_____ame	_____ane	_____eek
_____ool	_____ame	_____ane	_____eek
_____ool	_____ame	_____ane	_____eek
_____ool	_____ame	_____ane	_____eek
_____ool	_____ame	_____ane	_____eek

_____ook	_____ace	_____ape	_____eat
_____ook	_____ace	_____ape	_____eat
_____ook	_____ace	_____ape	_____eat
_____ook	_____ace	_____ape	_____eat
_____ook	_____ace	_____ape	_____eat

_____oot	_____ade	_____are	_____eal
_____oot	_____ade	_____are	_____eal
_____oot	_____ade	_____are	_____eal
_____oot	_____ade	___ __are	_____eal
_____oot	_____ade	_____are	_____eal

_____ore	_____age	_____ate	_____eed
_____ore	_____age	_____ate	_____eed
_____ore	_____age	_____ate	_____eed
_____ore	_____age	_____ate	_____eed
_____ore	_____age	_____ate	_____eed

100 items

FILL IN THE BLANK (INITIAL CONSONANT)

____ain	____ike	____ime	____ing
____ain	____ike	____ime	____ing
____ain	____ike	____ime	____ing
____ain	____ike	____ime	____ing
____ain	____ike	____ime	____ing
____ob	____ice	____ire	____est
____ob	____ice	____ire	____est
____ob	____ice	____ire	____est
____ob	____ice	____ire	____est
____ob	____ice	____ire	____est
____air	____ide	____ight	____oss
____air	____ide	____ight	____oss
____air	____ide	____ight	____oss
____air	____ide	____ight	____oss
____air	____ide	____ight	____oss
____old	____ind	____ive	____elt
____old	____ind	____ive	____elt
____old	____ind	____ive	____elt
____old	____ind	____ive	____elt
____old	____ind	____ive	____elt
____ine	____ile	____aid	____atch
____ine	____ile	____aid	____atch
____ine	____ile	____aid	____atch
____ine	____ile	____aid	____atch
____ine	____ile	____aid	____atch

100 items

FILL IN THE BLANK (INITIAL CONSONANT)

____at	____all	____am	____ar
____at	____all	____am	____ar
____at	____all	____am	____ar
____at	____all	____am	____ar
____at	____all	____am	____ar
____an	____ail	____ug	____ay
____an	____ail	____ug	____ay
____an	____ail	____ug	____ay
____an	____ail	____ug	____ay
____an	____ail	____ug	____ay
____un	____et	____ill	____og
____un	____et	____ill	____og
____un	____et	____ill	____og
____un	____et	____ill	____og
____un	____et	____ill	____og
____in	____ot	____ell	____ip
____in	____ot	____ell	____ip
____in	____ot	____ell	____ip
____in	____ot	____ell	____ip
____in	____ot	____ell	____ip
____ad	____ig	____ear	____ap
____ad	____ig	____ear	____ap
____ad	____ig	____ear	____ap
____ad	____ig	____ear	____ap
____ad	____ig	____ear	____ap

100 items

FILL IN THE BLANK (INITIAL CONSONANT OR BLEND)

____ack	____ump	____eep	____ipper
____ack	____ump	____eep	____ipper
____ack	____ump	____eep	____ipper
____ack		____eep	
	____y		____ar
____in	____y		____ar
____in	____y	____aw	
____in		____aw	
____in		____aw	____one
	____ay		____one
	____ay	____at	____one
____ew	____ay	____at	
____ew		____at	
____ew			____ap
	____op		____ap
	____op	____unk	____ap
____ick	____op	____unk	____ap
____ick	____op	____unk	
____ick			
____ick			____un
____ick	____am	____ink	____un
	____am	____ink	____un
	____am	____ink	____un
____ip			
____ip			
____ip	____amp	____ore	____ill
____ip	____amp	____ore	____ill
		____ore	____ill
		____ore	
____ock	____est		
____ock	____est		____ale
____ock	____est	____ave	____ale
____ock		____ave	____ale
		____ave	
	____ug		
____an	____ug		
____an		____erry	
____an		____erry	
	____um	____erry	
	____um		

100 items

FILL IN THE BLANK (INITIAL BLENDS)

____am	____in	____ate	____oop
____am	____in	____ate	____oop
____am	____in	____ate	____oop
____am	____in		
____am			
____am		____are	____ing
	____ake	____are	____ing
	____ake	____are	____ing
____an	____ake	____are	____ing
____an	____ake	____are	____ing
____an	____ake		
____an		____ip	____ash
	____ell	____ip	____ash
____and	____ell	____ip	____ash
____and	____ell	____ip	____ash
____and			____ash
____and			____ash
	____ed	____ide	____ash
____ick	____ed	____ide	
____ick	____ed	____ide	____at
____ick	____ed		____at
____ick	____ed		____at
____ick	____ed	____eet	____at
		____eet	____at
	____ack	____eet	____at
____im	____ack	____eet	
____im	____ack	____eet	
____im	____ack		____eam
____im	____ack	____eer	____eam
	____ack	____eer	____eam
	____ack	____eer	____eam
____oom		____eer	
____oom			
____oom			

100 items

FILL IN THE BLANK (INITIAL BLENDS)

____ain	____ip	____y	____ue
____ain	____ip	____y	____ue
____ain	____ip	____y	____ue
____ain	____ip	____y	
____ain	____ip	____y	
		____y	____ew
			____ew
____op	____ap		____ew
____op	____ap	____ing	____ew
____op	____ap	____ing	____ew
____op	____ap	____ing	
____op	____ap		____ee
		____air	____ee
____ag	____at	____air	____ee
____ag	____at	____air	
____ag	____at		____ow
____ag	____at	____ave	____ow
____ag	____at	____ave	____ow
		____ave	____ow
____ock	____ay	____ave	____ow
____ock	____ay	____ave	
____ock	____ay		____ot
____ock	____ay	____ill	____ot
____ock	____ay	____ill	____ot
		____ill	____ot
____ore	____ade	____ill	____ot
____ore	____ade	____ill	
____ore	____ade		
____ore	____ade	____ine	
____ore	____ade	____ine	
		____ine	
	____oke	____ine	
	____oke		
	____oke		

100 items

FILL IN THE BLANK (FINAL CONSONANT)

pu____	mu____	ja____	mo____
pu____	mu____	ja____	mo____
pu____	mu____	ja____	mo____
pu____		ja____	mo____
pu____			
	gu____		
	gu____	ga____	gri____
to____	gu____	ga____	gri____
to____		ga____	gri____
to____		ga____	gri____
to____	la____	ga____	gri____
to____	la____		
	la____		
	la____	ru____	bra____
no____	la____	ru____	bra____
no____		ru____	bra____
no____		ru____	bra____
no____	do____	ru____	
	do____		
	do____		sli____
pa____		le____	sli____
pa____		le____	sli____
pa____	na____	le____	sli____
pa____	na____	le____	
pa____	na____		
	Na____		sla____
		dra____	sla____
ro____		dra____	sla____
ro____	tri____	dra____	sla____
ro____	tri____		sla____
		sta____	
fla____	gra____	sta____	cla____
fla____	gra____	sta____	cla____
fla____		sta____	cla____
fla____			cla____
fla____			

100 items

FILL IN THE BLANK (FINAL CONSONANT)

co____	ra____	di____	bu____
co____	ra____	di____	bu____
co____	ra____	di____	bu____
co____	ra____	di____	bu____
co____	ra____		
		fa____	cu____
bi____	ca____	fa____	cu____
bi____	ca____	fa____	cu____
bi____	ca____	fa____	cu____
bi____	ca____		
bi____		ha____	be____
	si____	ha____	be____
wa____	si____	ha____	be____
wa____	si____	ha____	be____
wa____	si____		
		li____	da____
ba____	sa____	li____	da____
ba____	sa____	li____	da____
ba____	sa____		da____
ba____	sa____		
		ma____	fi____
ta____	ri____	ma____	fi____
ta____	ri____	ma____	fi____
ta____	ri____	ma____	fi____
ta____	ri____	ma____	fi____
ta____	ri____		
ta____		bo____	
	he____	bo____	hi____
jo____	he____	bo____	hi____
jo____	he____		hi____
jo____			hi____
			hi____

100 items

FILL IN THE BLANK (FINAL BLENDS)

ma____	wa____	wi____	li____
ma____	wa____	wi____	li____
ma____	wa____	wi____	li____
ma____	wa____	wi____	li____
ma____	wa____	wi____	li____
ma____	wa____		
	wa____		
		ri____	fa____
mi____		ri____	fa____
mi____	ba____	ri____	fa____
mi____	ba____	ri____	fa____
mi____	ba____	ri____	
mi____	ba____		
			mu____
		be____	mu____
a____	ba____	be____	mu____
a____	ba____	be____	
a____	ba____	be____	
a____	ba____		si____
a____			si____
		fo____	si____
	la____	fo____	si____
ha____	la____	fo____	
ha____	la____	fo____	
ha____	la____	fo____	wo____
ha____			wo____
ha____			wo____
ha____	bo____	co____	wo____
	bo____	co____	wo____
	bo____	co____	
	bo____	co____	
sa____	bo____	co____	we____
sa____		co____	we____
sa____			we____
sa____			
sa____			

100 items

FILL IN THE BLANK (SHORT VOWEL)

m___st	m___sh	j___g	t___n
m___st	m___sh	j___g	t___n
m___st	m___sh	j___g	t___n
		j___g	
sl___p	l___mp		h___tch
sl___p	l___mp	r___m	h___tch
sl___p	l___mp	r___m	h___tch
		r___m	
fl___p	t___ck		r___st
fl___p	t___ck	r___b	r___st
fl___p	t___ck	r___b	
	t___ck	r___b	st___ck
ch___p			st___ck
ch___p	l___st	r___g	st___ck
ch___p	l___st	r___g	st___ck
	l___st	r___g	
sl___m	l___st		b___nd
sl___m	l___st	r___mp	b___nd
sl___m		r___mp	b___nd
	r___ng	r___mp	
tr___ck	r___ng		f___t
tr___ck	r___ng	s___t	f___t
tr___ck		s___t	
	___n	s___t	v___t
w___g	___n		v___t
w___g	___n	t___g	
		t___g	___nd
s___ng	p___nt	t___g	___nd
s___ng	p___nt		
s___ng	p___nt	l___g	sp___n
s___ng		l___g	sp___n
	p___st	l___g	sp___n
	p___st	l___g	

100 items

FILL IN THE BLANK (SHORT VOWEL)

b___g	m___ss	p___t	p___p
b___g	m___ss	p___t	p___p
b___g	m___ss	p___t	p___p
b___g	m___ss	p___t	p___p
b___g	m___ss	p___t	
			l___t
g___t	d___ll	f___n	l___t
g___t	d___ll	f___n	l___t
g___t	d___ll	f___n	
	d___ll		l___ck
t___p		h___m	l___ck
t___p	f___ll	h___m	l___ck
t___p	f___ll	h___m	l___ck
	f___ll	h___m	
	f___ll		
c___p			d___ck
c___p		l___d	d___ck
c___p	b___ll	l___d	d___ck
	b___ll	l___d	d___ck
	b___ll		
p___ck	b___ll		l___st
p___ck		p___n	l___st
p___ck		p___n	l___st
p___ck	b___t	p___n	l___st
	b___t	p___n	l___st
	b___t		
n___t	b___t	l___ss	h___t
n___t		l___ss	h___t
n___t		l___ss	h___t
	r___d		h___t
	r___d		
h___t	r___d	d___g	
h___t		d___g	
h___t		d___g	s___ck
h___t			s___ck
			s___ck
s___x			s___ck
s___x			

100 items

FILL IN THE BLANK (LONG VOWEL)

b___ke	l___ce	t___me	l___te
b___ke	l___ce	t___me	l___te
w___de	s___le	t___ne	r___pe
w___de	s___le	t___ne	r___pe
		t___ne	r___pe
d___ve	c___ne		
d___ve	c___ne	f___me	tr___ce
		f___me	tr___ce
r___te	c___pe	f___ne	
r___te	c___pe		br___ke
r___te		d___me	br___ke
	m___le	d___me	
c___te	m___le	d___me	wr___te
k___te	m___le		wr___te
	m___le	d___ne	
p___ne		d___ne	fl___ke
p___ne	h___le		fl___ke
p___ne	h___le	b___ne	
		b___ne	sp___ce
m___te	w___'ve		sp___ce
m___te	w___ve	l___me	
m___te	w___ve	l___me	gr___pe
m___te	w___ves		gr___pe
		l___ne	gr___pe
___se	wh___le	l___ne	
___ce	wh___le	l___ne	sh___ne
___ce			sh___ne
	l___ke	r___se	
m___ce	l___ke	r___se	sp___ke
m___ce			sp___ke
	w___ne	r___ce	
c___ke	w___ne	r___ce	ph___se
c___ke			ph___ne
r___de			
r___de			
r___de			

100 items

SECTION 6: SENTENCES - CIRCLE THE WORD

<u>Directions</u>: Student reads orally the entire sheet. Teacher reads the first sentence orally and says one of the underlined words incorrectly. The student circles the word he heard that was pronounced incorrectly. The teacher proceeds to read the next sentence, etc.

<u>Example</u>: The <u>fat</u> <u>cat</u> chased a <u>rat</u>.

> Teacher reads the sentence in a manner such as this:

>> "The fat mat chased a rat."
>> or
>> "The fat rabbit chased a rat."

> The student circles one word he heard the teacher say incorrectly.

> The <u>answer</u>:

>> The <u>fat</u> <u>cat</u> chased a <u>rat</u>.

SENTENCES - CIRCLE THE WORD

1. The man liked to jog with the dog in the fog.

2. Heather wore leather boots in snowy weather.

3. Herman heard a sermon in German.

4. The clown with the brown nose went to town.

5. Sometimes Hester and Esther like to pester the animals at the zoo.

6. The king liked to swing and sing.

7. Vince, the prince, liked mince meat pie.

8. The hare and the bear shared a ripe pear.

9. The seal skated with zeal on a banana peel.

10. Joe put new snow tires on his tow truck.

11. Lance, a native of France, performed a lovely dance.

12. Some Quakers were bakers and some were cabinet makers.

13. Her face lit up when she saw the vase and the new lace for her gown.

14. He put his pet duck in the truck for good luck.

15. The boy who plays a horn was born in a cornfield.

16. The stork ate some pork with a fork.

17. Dale, the whale, swallowed a nail.

18. The grand old band marched in the sand.

19. Sam liked to eat jam and clams.

20. Chad was glad to wear his plaid suit.

21. Billy and Willy acted funny and silly.

22. Ned put his sled in the shed.

23. Peter studied about the meter and the liter.

24. Kenny and Denny found a rare penny.

25. Mr. Weed took a class to learn to speed read.

25 items

SENTENCES - CIRCLE THE WORD

1. I will go to the show with Joe.

2. Mother will bake a cake to take to the picnic.

3. That big dog sat on my new hat.

4. One dark night we heard a dog bark in the park.

5. Where is the bear who ate my pear?

6. I was kind to the blind man when I helped him find his good dog.

7. The teacher gave a thumb tack to Mack who sat in the back of the room.

8. Since Mother had to go to town, Joe had to mow the lawn.

9. Dad was sad and very mad.

10. Jim and Tim knew they would win the game.

11. Pete grew wheat in his garden and got meat from his cows.

12. If I could drive a car I would, but I don't think I should.

13. I found my hound at the dog pound.

14. I thought the man with the gun shot Scott.

15. Someone lost a clock, a sock, and a piece of chalk.

16. Who put glue in my new shoe?

17. I gave the nice mice some rice to eat.

18. When we dropped the bell we had to tell Mrs. Well, our principal.

19. See the bee hive in the big tree.

20. The man lived in a house near the pier for almost a year.

21. The witch fell in the ditch because she had a bad itch.

22. Snow White had to sew for the seven dwarfs and grow plants in a garden.

23. When you hear the bell chime, I'll give you a dime if you say a rhyme.

24. The poor man wore a torn coat and had no more food left in his house.

25. When did the men find the ten horses?

25 items

SENTENCES - CIRCLE THE WORD

1. One <u>sunny</u> day I saw a <u>funny</u> white <u>bunny</u>.

2. <u>Ted</u> <u>said</u> that he <u>read</u> the book.

3. I <u>wish</u> that I could eat a <u>dish</u> of <u>fish</u>.

4. <u>Bill</u> and <u>Jill</u> fell down the <u>hill</u>.

5. After <u>lunch</u> we like to <u>munch</u> on a <u>bunch</u> of grapes.

6. When <u>Ben</u> was <u>ten</u> years old he got a <u>hen</u>.

7. The <u>cold</u> man <u>told</u> me that he <u>sold</u> his dog.

8. <u>Rick</u> got <u>sick</u> when we went to <u>pick</u> berries.

9. I <u>let</u> my <u>pet</u> kitten take a ride on a <u>jet</u> airplane.

10. <u>Ned</u> bumped his <u>head</u> on his <u>bed</u>.

11. The <u>fat</u> <u>cat</u> chased a <u>rat</u>.

12. We went to <u>see</u> <u>Lee</u> when <u>he</u> was in the hospital.

13. We had to <u>stop</u> at the <u>shop</u> to get some bottles of <u>pop</u>.

14. <u>Please</u> get the <u>bees</u> and <u>fleas</u> out of this garage.

15. On the first <u>day</u> of <u>May</u> the children were happy and <u>gay</u>.

16. <u>Burt</u> wore a red <u>shirt</u> and Jane wore a red <u>skirt</u>.

17. <u>Dick</u> gave the ball a <u>quick</u> <u>kick</u>.

18. <u>Paul</u> got a <u>ball</u> for Christmas and Sally got a <u>doll</u>.

19. Let's <u>try</u> a piece of <u>my</u> lemon <u>pie</u>.

20. I saw the airplane <u>fly</u> <u>high</u> up in the <u>sky</u>.

21. I wore a heavy <u>coat</u> on the <u>boat</u> ride because I had a sore <u>throat</u>.

22. The <u>king</u> with a big <u>ring</u> on his finger asked the people to <u>sing</u>.

23. The <u>cute</u> little boy in the brown <u>suit</u> played a <u>flute</u>.

24. The <u>goose</u> and the <u>moose</u> liked to drink grape <u>juice</u>.

25. <u>You</u> saw <u>two</u> tigers at the <u>zoo</u>.

25 items

Directions: The student reads orally the entire sheet. The teacher says orally a sentence for each item on the page including the number answer. The student writes the number he heard beside the corresponding item. Do not say items in order. Answers can range from one to thousands, dollars and cents, and even fractions. A teacher can be very creative in this section.

Example:

1. Teacher says, "Jane was born at 8:12 a.m." Student writes 8:12 a.m. in the blank next to Jane. Answer: Jane 8:12 a.m.

2. Teacher says, "The apples cost $5.28." Student writes what he heard in the blank next to apples. Answer: apples $5.28.

3. Teacher says, "Joe's license number is 621-375." (Alphabet letters can be used here, also.) Student writes what he heard in the blank next to Joe. Answer: Joe 621-375.

4. Teacher says, "It was 85 degrees on Flag Day." Student writes what he heard in the blank next to Flag Day. Answer: Flag Day 85°.

Another method for sections 7 and 9 is: The student asks a question about each item on the sheet. The teacher responds with a sentence answer. This method is less difficult.

Example:

1. Student asks, "What is Jane's telephone number?" Teacher answers, "Jane's telephone number is 855-6213." Student writes what he heard next to Jane. Answer: Jane 855-6213.

2. Student asks, "What musical instrument did Sally play?" Teacher answers, "Sally played an oboe." Student writes Sally's number in the blank beside oboe. Answer: 1. Joe _____ drum
2. Moe 3 oboe
3. Sally _____ trumpet

70

WHAT ARE THEIR AGES?

Jane_____   Judy_____   Kay_____   Sherry_____

John_____   Christy_____   Wally_____   Jerry_____

Joan_____   Missy_____   Sally_____   Tommy_____

Jean_____   Rita_____   Lilly_____   Timmy_____

Janis_____   Penny_____   Willy_____   Tammy_____

Julie_____   Dave_____   Larry_____   Betty_____

Joe_____   Ray_____   Gary_____   Amy_____

James_____   Lee_____   Harry_____   Kathy_____

Joy_____

33 items

HOW MANY PETS WERE IN THE PET STORE?

dogs_____   mice_____   frogs_____

cats_____   monkeys_____   toads_____

chickens_____   snakes_____   butterflies_____

hamsters_____   lizards_____   hens_____

bunnies_____   kittens_____   turkeys_____

ducks_____   puppies_____   peacocks_____

turtles_____   rabbits_____   eagles_____

fish_____   donkeys_____   robins_____

poodles_____   sheep_____   goats_____

ponies_____   lambs_____   goldfish_____

horses_____   roosters_____   zebras_____

33 items

HOW MANY OF EACH ITEM DID THEY PURCHASE

AT THE GROCERY STORE?

____bread	____corn	____soap	____jelly
____butter	____cereal	____tissue	____peanuts
____cheese	____bacon	____salt	____margarine
____eggs	____cake	____pepper	____jello
____milk	____pie	____beans	____pudding
____apples	____fish	____steaks	____cookies
____oranges	____soup	____chicken	____ice cream
____bananas	____crackers	____melons	____ham
____plums	____spaghetti	____carrots	____crabs
____pears	____peppers	____oil	____mustard
____peaches	____tomatoes	____vinegar	____pickles
____lettuce	____potatoes	____candy	____ketchup
____peas			____gum

50 items

WHAT WAS THE TEMPERATURE ON THESE DAYS?

Christmas_____   Flag Day_____

Hanukkah_____   Father's Day_____

New Year's Eve_____   Labor Day_____

New Year's Day_____   Independence Day_____

Ash Wednesday_____   Citizenship Day_____

Valentine's Day_____   Rosh Hashanah_____

Lincoln's Birthday_____   Yom Kippur_____

Washington's Birthday_____   Columbus Day_____

Easter_____   Halloween_____

Palm Sunday_____   United Nation's Day_____

Good Friday_____   Sweetest Day_____

St. Patrick's Day_____   Election Day_____

Passover_____   Veterans Day_____

Secretary's Day_____   Thanksgiving_____

Mother's Day_____   Earth Day_____

Memorial Day_____   April Fool's Day_____

                                        First Day of School_____

33 items

HOW TALL WERE THEY?

Mr. Jones_____   Mr. White_____

Mrs. Jones_____   Mrs. White_____

Miss Jones_____   Miss White_____

Master Jones_____   Master White_____

Doctor Jones_____   Doctor White_____

Mr. Stone_____   Reverend White_____

Mrs. Stone_____   Mr. Wright_____

Miss Stone_____   Mrs. Wright_____

Master Stone_____   Miss Wright_____

Doctor Stone_____   Master Wright_____

Mr. Post_____   Doctor Wright_____

Mrs. Post_____   Senator Wright_____

Miss Post_____   Mr. Stein_____

Master Post_____   Mrs. Stein_____

Doctor Post_____   Miss Stein_____

Professor Post_____   Master Stein_____

                                       Doctor Stein_____

33 items

HOW MUCH DO THEY WEIGH?

ham_____lbs._____oz.   asparagus_____lbs._____oz.

roast beef_____lbs._____oz.   corn_____lbs._____oz.

turkey_____lbs._____oz.   potatoes_____lbs._____oz.

chicken_____lbs._____oz.   yams_____lbs._____oz.

shrimp_____lbs._____oz.   squash_____lbs._____oz.

bananas_____lbs._____oz.   Joseph_____lbs._____oz.

apples_____lbs._____oz.   Valerie_____lbs._____oz.

tangerines_____lbs._____oz.   Nancy_____lbs._____oz.

limes_____lbs._____oz.   Simon_____lbs._____oz.

pears_____lbs._____oz.   Walter_____lbs._____oz.

                                           Alex_____lbs._____oz.

peanuts_____lbs._____oz.   Barbara_____lbs._____oz.

pecans_____lbs._____oz.   Gloria_____lbs._____oz.

walnuts_____lbs._____oz.

almonds_____lbs._____oz.   elephant_____lbs._____oz.

cashews_____lbs._____oz.   parakeet_____lbs._____oz.

                                           poodle_____lbs._____oz.

                                           Siamese cat_____lbs._____oz.

                                           German Shepherd_____lbs._____oz.

33 items

HOW MANY BOOKS OF TRADING STAMPS FOR EACH?

____watch	____ice bucket	____blackboard
____umbrella	____lawn mower	____playpen
____pearls	____bowling ball	____buggy
____mirror	____briefcase	____toaster
____stapler	____catcher's mitt	____coffeepot
____dictionary	____pillows	____iron
____typewriter	____camera	____steak knives
____luggage	____golf clubs	____can opener
____blanket	____clock	____picture
____rug	____skis	____rocking chair
____scale	____teapot	____card table
____sheets	____cookie jar	____organ
____basketball	____radio	____piano
____football	____color TV	____golf shoes
____tablecloth	____tape recorder	____ladder
____bedspread	____trumpet	____globe
____hair dryer	____bicycle	

50 items

WHAT TIME WERE THEY BORN?

Adam_____   Mary_____

Barney_____   Morgan_____

Calvin_____   Pauline_____

Dwight_____   Mabel_____

Ed_____   Jack_____

Ann_____   Jim_____

April_____   Joyce_____

Roger_____   James_____

Peter_____   Dixie_____

Oliver_____   Bill_____

Frank_____   Bob_____

Gregory_____   Louis_____

Elizabeth_____   Max_____

Violet_____   Leroy_____

Hazel_____   Glenn_____

Sally_____   Loretta_____

Valerie_____

33 items

WHAT ARE THEIR LICENSE NUMBERS?

Stephen_____   Tom_____

Kenny_____   Alice_____

Jeff_____   Bruce_____

Don_____   Danny_____

Bill_____   Jane_____

Dale_____   Carol_____

Ruth_____   Dennis_____

Lisa_____   Ann_____

Paul_____   Susan_____

Denise_____   Joe_____

Francis_____   Edward_____

Robert_____   Jim_____

John_____

25 items

TELEPHONE NUMBERS

Susan_____	Jack_____
Julie_____	Chuck_____
Christy_____	Duke_____
James_____	Daisy_____
David_____	Beth_____
Janis_____	Betty_____
Danny_____	Sammy_____
Steve_____	John_____
Robert_____	Judy_____
Jeff_____	Rudy_____
Christine_____	Lucy_____
Ruth_____	Janet_____
Luke_____	Patty_____
Missy_____	Greg_____
June_____	Robin_____
Hugh_____	Jean_____
Ted_____	

33 items

WHAT ARE THE PRICES?

lettuce_____	grapes_____
celery_____	apples_____
parsley_____	pears_____
peppers_____	peaches_____
squash_____	plums_____
cabbage_____	oranges_____
carrots_____	bananas_____
turnips_____	cherries_____
parsnips_____	cantaloupes_____
radishes_____	strawberries_____
corn_____	avocados_____
onions_____	blueberries_____
potatoes_____	tangerines_____
tomatoes_____	watermelons_____
spinach_____	blackberries_____
broccoli_____	pineapples_____
endive_____	

33 items

Directions: Student reads orally the entire page. Teacher says a phrase. According to what the student heard, he marks a number from an item on the page in a blank beside the item that goes with it.

Example:

   1. pink   <u> 2 </u> kite
   2. blue   <u>   </u> bike
   3. purple   <u>   </u> knife

Teacher says, "A blue kite." Student writes the number beside "blue" in the blank next to what he heard.

Example:

   1. Your   <u> 1 </u> camel
   2. Our   <u>   </u> candle
   3. His   <u> 2 </u> castle

Teacher says, "Our castle." Student writes number 2 beside CASTLE. Teacher says,""Your camel." Student writes number 1 beside CAMEL.

COLORS I

1. pink	5. white	9. black	13. gray
2. blue	6. green	10. brown	14. navy
3. purple	7. yellow	11. orange	15. beige
4. gold	8. red	12. silver	16. tan

____kite	____rake	____sheet	____room
____bike	____lake	____string	____book
____knife	____lace	____boot	____coat
____tie	____leaf	____shoe	____boat
____pipe	____tree	____suit	____rose
____cane	____ring	____broom	____soap
____cake			

25 items

COLORS II

1. rust	5. coral	8. rose	11. ivory
2. violet	6. lemon	9. maroon	12. mauve
3. lime	7. wine	10. aqua	13. taupe
4. olive			

____hat	____desk	____pants	____stain
____cat	____plaque	____slacks	____vase
____mat	____cast	____drapes	____frame
____flask	____tam	____plate	____case
____cap	____clasp	____shake	____lace
____vest	____patch	____cape	____lake
____mask			

25 items

ADJECTIVES

1. Your	4. Her
2. Our	5. My
3. His	6. Their

____camel   ____rattle   ____pistol   ____daughter

____candle   ____whistle   ____paddle   ____pocket

____castle   ____fiddle   ____butter   ____locket

____cattle   ____pickle   ____father   ____rocket

____saddle   ____nickel   ____feather   ____basket

____sandle   ____bottle   ____heather   ____chocolate

____gavel

25 items

ADJECTIVES

1. dreary	8. worried	14. locked	20. rotted
2. cherry	9. weary	15. soft	21. dotted
3. merry	10. blueberry	16. lost	22. knotted
4. berry	11. strawberry	17. chopped	23. spotted
5. dairy	12. raspberry	18. tossed	24. frosted
6. fairy	13. blackberry	19. huckleberry	25. potted
7. hairy			

____teacher	____rat	____pie	____dog
____doctor	____sundae	____door	____tart
____salad	____Monday	____child	____ham
____tale	____jam	____vest	____ice cream
____farm	____jelly	____plant	____cake
____widow	____preserves	____pipe	____rope
____wine			

25 items

ADJECTIVES

1. sly	8. wise	14. rear	20. fast
2. shy	9. fair	15. poor	21. last
3. rye	10. flared	16. sore	22. brass
4. dry	11. clear	17. torn	23. true
5. kind	12. dear	18. worn	24. new
6. pine	13. feared	19. vast	25. blue
7. nice			

____desert	____fox	____husband	____story
____owl	____arm	____trumpet	____woman
____family	____test	____seat	____horse
____glass	____diamond	____spray	____leg
____day	____bread	____people	____horn
____skirt	____policeman	____sheet	____eyes
____wife			

25 items

ADJECTIVES

1. funny	8. fuzzy	14. misty	20. cloudy
2. sunny	9. dizzy	15. witty	21. happy
3. yummy	10. busy	16. crispy	22. silly
4. lumpy	11. frizzy	17. slippery	23. fancy
5. lazy	12. nippy	18. mushy	24. husky
6. hazy	13. tasty	19. dreamy	25. windy
7. crazy			

____clown	____bee	____bear	____music
____sandwich	____snow	____cereal	____baby
____sky	____afternoon	____hose	____boxer
____hair	____toast	____goose	____beach
____clouds	____student	____bunny	____celery
____sidewalk	____morning	____street	____oats
____evening			

25 items

ADJECTIVES

1. light	8. gold	14. glad	20. sweet
2. bright	9. cold	15. lean	21. neat
3. right	10. bad	16. clean	22. smart
4. tight	11. sad	17. teen	23. tart
5. white	12. mad	18. mean	24. dark
6. old	13. plaid	19. cream	25. fat
7. bold			

____pie	____dress	____desk	____child
____skirt	____king	____kitten	____car
____giant	____woman	____teacher	____soda
____girl	____teeth	____cake	____doctor
____house	____ice cream	____crown	____father
____baby	____queen	____closet	____coat
____attic			

25 items

ADJECTIVES

1. western	8. heather	14. pork	20. storm
2. nice	9. better	15. corn	21. smart
3. tidy	10. bitter	16. cork	22. sharp
4. ripe	11. icy	17. coarse	23. hard
5. striped	12. slimy	18. foreign	24. torn
6. white	13. short	19. dark	25. worn
7. leather			

____Christmas   ____shadow   ____roll   ____cheese

____bread   ____dress   ____shoe   ____paper

____window   ____roast   ____lizard   ____weather

____purse   ____person   ____grape   ____couch

____bridge   ____floor   ____field   ____car

____banana   ____hair   ____room   ____pupil

____movie

25 items

SECTION 9: SENTENCES

Directions: Student reads orally the entire page to assure correct pronunciation of each word. Definitions may be discussed, also, if student
is not familiar with the meanings of all the words. Teacher says a sentence. According to what the student heard, he marks a number from an
item on the page in a blank beside the item that goes with it.

Example: What Did They Hear?

   1. Matt   2 bells
   2. Pat   3 rain
   3. cat   1 thunder

Teacher says, "Matt heard thunder." Student writes a number 1 beside
THUNDER. Teacher says, "The cat heard rain." Student writes a number 3
beside RAIN.

WHAT DID THEY HAVE?

1. Boy	8. Rhoda	14. Warren	20. Wayne
2. Tony	9. Tarzan	15. Marty	21. Shane
3. Toby	10. Barbara	16. Marcy	22. Jane
4. Joey	11. Nora	17. Mark	23. Mame
5. Jody	12. Martha	18. Charlotte	24. Dave
6. Moe	13. Marsha	19. Dwayne	25. Steve
7. Joe			

____party	____cold	____toothache	____sister
____picnic	____test	____appointment	____brother
____wreck	____fever	____headache	____friend
____lunch	____secret	____argument	____baby
____dinner	____accident	____snack	____date
____breakfast	____fight	____homework	____dream
____fun			

WHAT DID THEY MAKE?

1. Marlene	8. Sharon	14. Martha	20. Ray
2. Darlene	9. Mary	15. Marsha	21. Babe
3. Arlene	10. Jerry	16. Tarzan	22. Abe
4. Sharlene	11. Laura	17. Jane	23. Gabe
5. Karen	12. Carla	18. Stan	24. Jimmy
6. Carolyn	13. Carl	19. Wayne	25. Ginny
7. Darren			

_____cake	_____sweater	_____salad	_____homerun
_____pie	_____mistake	_____bread	_____choice
_____dress	_____error	_____friend	_____decision
_____skirt	_____popcorn	_____pizza	_____incision
_____pillow	_____appointment	_____enemy	_____right turn
_____rug	_____bed	_____touchdown	_____U turn
_____wish			

25 items

WHAT DID THEY HEAR?

1. Matt	8. turtle	14. he	20. Norris
2. Pat	9. dog	15. she	21. Bunny
3. cat	10. bee	16. horse	22. Sonny
4. rat	11. we	17. Boris	23. Penny
5. monkey	12. Lee	18. Doris	24. Denny
6. donkey	13. Dee	19. Nora	25. Wendy
7. bird			

____bells	____helicopter	____band	____singing
____rain	____motor boat	____whistle	____airplane
____thunder	____music	____horns	____train
____storm	____radio	____siren	____telephone
____lawn mower	____tape recorder	____laughing	____wind
____dishwasher	____television	____cheering	____drum
____traffic			

25 items

WHAT MUSICAL INSTRUMENTS DID THEY PLAY?

1. Dad	8. Nell	14. Ron	20. Helen
2. Tad	9. Will	15. Fran	21. Max
3. Chad	10. Hal	16. Jan	22. Rex
4. Dot	11. Tom	17. Stan	23. Tex
5. Scott	12. Mom	18. Pam	24. Beth
6. Gale	13. Don	19. Ellen	25. Wes
7. Dale			

____piano	____trumpet	____saxophone	____tambourine
____organ	____French horn	____snare drum	____viola
____flute	____trombone	____bongo drum	____cello
____harp	____clarinet	____guitar	____harpsichord
____violin	____fiddle	____harmonica	____cornet
____drum	____piccolo	____oboe	____accordion
____cymbals			

25 items

WHAT WERE THEY ON HALLOWEEN?

1. Jay	8. he	14. Ray	20. Lou
2. May	9. she	15. Jane	21. Sue
3. Gay	10. Vee	16. James	22. Drew
4. Kay	11. Lee	17. Bruce	23. Trudy
5. Fay	12. Jean	18. Lucy	24. Judy
6. Dee	13. Jake	19. June	25. Susie
7. Bea			

____witch   ____fortune teller   ____rabbit   ____Indian

____pumpkin   ____ballerina   ____tramp   ____clown

____bat   ____tiger   ____bride   ____cowboy

____ghost   ____bull dog   ____queen   ____pilgrim

____gypsy   ____cat   ____princess   ____devil

____astronaut   ____monster   ____knight   ____football
                                                            player

____pirate

25 items

WHAT WERE THEIR NATIONALITIES?

1. Hilda	8. Millie	14. Zelda	20. Helen
2. Wilma	9. Lily	15. Melba	21. Velma
3. Bill	10. Gilda	16. Ellie	22. Thelma
4. Jill	11. Delia	17. Nellie	23. Elmer
5. Phillip	12. Celia	18. Belle	24. Selma
6. Milton	13. Tilly	19. Dale	25. Della
7. Willie			

____Russian   ____Scottish   ____French   ____Chinese

____American   ____Danish   ____Roman   ____Japanese

____Mexican   ____Dutch   ____Swiss   ____Greek

____Italian   ____Polish   ____Welsh   ____Jewish

____German   ____Canadian   ____Korean   ____Indian

____Australian   ____Spanish   ____Irish   ____Swedish

____English

25 items

WHAT TREES DID THEY PLANT?

1. Laura	8. Jerry	14. Jordan	20. Ivan
2. Sara	9. Gerald	15. Forest	21. Clyde
3. Darrin	10. Harold	16. Morton	22. Guy
4. Erin	11. Farrah	17. Norton	23. Ira
5. Sharon	12. Boris	18. Iris	24. Lila
6. Carol	13. Doris	19. Dinah	25. Milo
7. Gary			

____fir	____chestnut	____spruce	____poplar
____pine	____cypress	____hemlock	____boxwood
____oak	____maple	____ash	____ebony
____cedar	____hickory	____locust	____beech
____birch	____elm	____magnolia	____aspen
____teak	____willow	____redwood	____yew
____walnut			

25 items

WHAT DID THEY PLANT IN THEIR GARDENS?

1. Marcy	8. Tara	14. Lori	20. Penny
2. Marty	9. Larry	15. Corey	21. Cindy
3. Gary	10. Chrissy	16. Porky	22. Linda
4. Harry	11. Missy	17. Corky	23. Benny
5. Sherry	12. Sissy	18. Norma	24. Sonny
6. Terry	13. Patty	19. Lorna	25. Bunny
7. Sara			

____roses
____daisies
____tomatoes
____potatoes
____peppers
____mums
____corn

____tulips
____bluebells
____blueberries
____strawberries
____cherries
____grapes

____parsley
____violets
____lilies
____pumpkins
____pom poms
____cabbage

____celery
____lettuce
____onions
____pears
____peaches
____apples

25 items

WHAT DID THEY OPEN?

1. Emma	8. Ted	14. Karen	20. Steve
2. Emily	9. Chet	15. Joe	21. Jean
3. Amy	10. Chester	16. Hope	22. Kay
4. Esther	11. Betsy	17. Jody	23. Jay
5. Fred	12. Kent	18. Eve	24. May
6. Beth	13. Kevin	19. Lee	25. Wayne
7. Ned			

____box	____letter	____magazine	____refrigerator
____door	____package	____purse	____dishwasher
____jar	____mail	____locker	____briefcase
____closet	____can	____safe	____cupboard
____drawer	____bottle	____mailbox	____jewelry box
____gift	____suitcase	____oven	____pocketbook
____present			

25 items

WHAT FISH DID THEY EAT?

1. Jay	8. Dean	14. Scott	20. Mom
2. Wade	9. Jean	15. Dot	21. John
3. Jade	10. Pete	16. Don	22. Jenny
4. May	11. Eve	17. Tom	23. Benny
5. Fay	12. Steve	18. Paul	24. Denny
6. they	13. Tate	19. Saul	25. Wendy
7. Wayne			

____catfish	____bluefish	____halibut	____salmon
____trout	____eel	____red snapper	____sardines
____sole	____herring	____whiting	____pike
____perch	____haddock	____grouper	____spots
____flounder	____turbot	____swordfish	____pompano
____cod	____scrod	____tuna	____dolphin
____whitefish			

25 items

WHAT DID THEY STUDY?

1. Lisa	6. Dean	11. James	16. Morris
2. Leah	7. Jean	12. Wayne	17. Doris
3. Lee	8. Pete	13. Layne	18. Boris
4. Rita	9. Amy	14. Mame	19. Forrest
5. Frieda	10. Jamie	15. Dave	20. Grace

____Language Arts

____Math

____Social Studies

____Science

____Spelling

____American History

____World Cultures

____French

____German

____Spanish

____Literature

____Poetry

____Biology

____Chemistry

____English

____Music

____Geometry

____Art

____Algebra

____Speech

20 items

WHAT BIRDS DID THEY SEE?

1. Sue	8. May	14. Peter	20. Eddie
2. Drew	9. Ray	15. Jack	21. Betty
3. Lou	10. June	16. Matt	22. Wendy
4. Ruth	11. Dean	17. Pat	23. Sandy
5. Jane	12. Stephen	18. Stan	24. Fanny
6. Kay	13. Lisa	19. Debbie	25. Danny
7. Fay			

____bluebird	____owl	____falcon	____catbird
____finch	____robin	____flamingo	____sparrow
____thrush	____wren	____peacock	____mockingbird
____buzzard	____cardinal	____bluejay	____crane
____crow	____cuckoo	____canary	____nightingale
____hawk	____lark	____parrot	____woodpecker
____flicker			

25 items

WHERE DID THEY GO ON THEIR VACATIONS?

1. Ann	8. Lou	14. Flo	20. Nell
2. Sam	9. Drew	15. Moe	21. Jane
3. Jim	10. Sue	16. Bill	22. Wayne
4. John	11. Hugh	17. Will	23. Amos
5. Dan	12. Joe	18. Phil	24. Tom
6. Nan	13. Rhoda	19. Jill	25. Rose
7. Pam			

_____New York   _____Maryland   _____South Carolina

_____Maine   _____Ohio   _____Kentucky

_____Vermont   _____Arizona   _____North Carolina

_____Texas   _____Alabama   _____Tennessee

_____Oregon   _____Montana   _____Missouri

_____New Mexico   _____Kansas   _____Indiana

_____Florida   _____New Jersey   _____Michigan

_____Georgia   _____Rhode Island   _____Oklahoma

_____Virginia

25 items

HOW DID THEY FEEL?

1. Mom	8. Ned	14. Vee	20. Mack
2. Tom	9. Ted	15. Dee	21. Jane
3. Ron	10. Ed	16. Bea	22. Zane
4. John	11. Matt	17. he	23. Mame
5. Don	12. Pat	18. she	24. Shane
6. Tad	13. Jack	19. Lee	25. Ava
7. Chad			

_____joyful

_____happy

_____content

_____tired

_____cold

_____warm

_____irritable

_____sorry

_____guilty

_____silly

_____embarrassed

_____sad

_____weak

_____ashamed

_____wonderful

_____foolish

_____proud

_____brave

_____scared

_____frightened

_____nervous

_____confident

_____depressed

_____enthusiastic

_____anxious

25 items

WHERE WERE THEY?

1. Joe	8. Jan	14. Bill	20. Patty
2. Sue	9. Jim	15. Pat	21. Hattie
3. Lou	10. John	16. Jack	22. Matty
4. Joan	11. Jane	17. Mack	23. Kathy
5. Ann	12. Tom	18. Dick	24. Mick
6. Dan	13. Bob	19. Rick	25. Nick
7. Sam			

____car	____garage	____movie	____pool
____bedroom	____playroom	____hospital	____barn
____school	____library	____dining room	____attic
____church	____outside	____upstairs	____camp
____park	____downstairs	____living room	____greenhouse
____zoo	____store	____garden	____apartment
____kitchen			

25 items

WHAT DID THEY READ?

1. Bart	8. Gill	14. Willy	20. Wilda
2. Art	9. Jill	15. Billy	21. Wilma
3. Clark	10. Shelley	16. Lynn	22. Hilda
4. Mark	11. Kelly	17. Glenn	23. Zelda
5. Bill	12. Nellie	18. Wynne	24. Selma
6. Neal	13. Lilly	19. Pam	25. Velma
7. Dale			

____magazine   ____encyclopedia   ____nursery rhyme   ____pamphlet

____novel   ____poem   ____research study   ____report

____mystery   ____play   ____riddle   ____speech

____newspaper   ____essay   ____libretto   ____cookbook

____dictionary   ____short story   ____comic strip   ____fairy tale

____Bible   ____sonnet   ____textbook   ____recipe

____newsletter

25 items

WHAT WERE THEIR FAVORITE SPORTS?

1. Stan	8. Van	14. Ron	20. Ned
2. Dan	9. Len	15. Tom	21. Jed
3. Ann	10. Sam	16. John	22. Fred
4. Fran	11. Jim	17. Ben	23. Red
5. Jan	12. Tim	18. Clem	24. Kim
6. Nan	13. Slim	19. Ted	25. Glenn
7. Pam			

____hockey   ____fishing   ____rowing

____tennis   ____ice skating   ____snow skiing

____swimming   ____golf   ____boat racing

____football   ____bowling   ____wrestling

____baseball   ____water skiing   ____boxing

____basketball   ____sailing   ____surfing

____volleyball   ____car racing   ____horseback riding

____soccer   ____softball

____hunting   ____archery

25 items

WHERE DO THE PETS LIVE?

1. Spot	8. Bunny	14. Brownie	20. Queenie
2. Top	9. Scotty	15. Fluffy	21. Tessie
3. Tip	10. Happy	16. King	22. Bessie
4. Skippy	11. Tabby	17. Tammy	23. Betsy
5. Boots	12. Blacky	18. Duke	24. Honey
6. Lassie	13. Whitey	19. Maggie	25. Missy
7. Hoppy			

____1st Street	____10th Street	____18th Street
____2nd Street	____11th Street	____19th Street
____3rd Street	____12th Street	____30th Street
____4th Street	____13th Street	____40th Street
____5th Street	____14th Street	____50th Street
____6th Street	____15th Street	____60th Street
____7th Street	____16th Street	____70th Street
____8th Street	____17th Street	____80th Street
____9th Street		

25 items

WHAT TEAMS DID THEY ROOT FOR?

1. Bill	8. Nell	14. Olin	20. Beau
2. Will	9. Neil	15. Gillian	21. Flo
3. Phil	10. Belle	16. Lillian	22. Joan
4. Gill	11. Ellen	17. William	23. Joy
5. Jill	12. Helen	18. Joe	24. Boyd
6. Lil	13. Allen	19. Moe	25. Roy
7. Mel			

_____Washington Redskins

_____St. Louis Cardinals

_____Pittsburgh Steelers

_____Miami Dolphins

_____Houston Oilers

_____New York Jets

_____Minnesota Vikings

_____Philadelphia Eagles

_____Denver Broncos

_____Detroit Lions

_____Cleveland Browns

_____Chicago Bears

_____Oakland Raiders

_____Seattle Seahawks

_____Buffalo Bills

_____Atlanta Falcons

_____Cincinnati Bengals

_____Los Angeles Rams

_____San Francisco 49ers

_____New Orleans Saints

_____New England Patriots

_____Baltimore Colts

_____Kansas City Chiefs

_____San Diego Chargers

_____Dallas Cowboys

25 items

WHAT STATE CAPITALS DID THEY VISIT?

1. Mike	8. Tiny	14. Beth	20. Pris
2. Iris	9. Clyde	15. Ken	21. Missy
3. Ivy	10. Dinah	16. Ben	22. Sissy
4. Ida	11. Lila	17. Fess	23. Chris
5. Irene	12. Wes	18. Tess	24. Chrissy
6. Myra	13. Bess	19. Len	25. Kristin
7. Guy			

____Charleston	____Columbia	____Jackson	____Atlanta
____Salem	____Albany	____Lansing	____Sacramento
____Boston	____Columbus	____Harrisburg	____Boise
____Honolulu	____Nashville	____Concord	____Austin
____Dover	____Helena	____Trenton	____Providence
____Annapolis	____Carson City	____Richmond	____Raleigh
____Salt Lake City			

25 items

TO WHAT ISLANDS DID THEY SAIL?

1. Mr. Dailey	10. Rev. Bailey	18. Mrs. Shale
2. Mrs. Dailey	11. Mr. Bell	19. Miss Shale
3. Miss Dailey	12. Mrs. Bell	20. Master Shale
4. Master Dailey	13. Miss Bell	21. Rev. Shale
5. Mr. Bailey	14. Master Bell	22. Mr. Kale
6. Mrs. Bailey	15. Dr. Bell	23. Mrs. Kale
7. Miss Bailey	16. Rev. Bell	24. Miss Kale
8. Master Bailey	17. Mr. Shale	25. Dr. Kale
9. Dr. Bailey		

____Bermuda

____Wake

____Guam

____Midway

____Capri

____Tahiti

____Haiti

____Hawaii

____Puerto Rico

____Bahamas

____St. Thomas

____St. John

____Jamaica

____Canary Islands

____St. Vincent

____Japan

____Bora Bora

____Java

____Cuba

____Greenland

____Iceland

____Taiwan

____Sicily

____Ireland

____Catalina

25 items

WHAT CHARACTERS DID THEY READ ABOUT?

1. Connie	8. Sandy	14. Frannie	20. Brad
2. Bonnie	9. Mandy	15. Granny	21. Dad
3. Donnie	10. Danny	16. Cappy	22. Lad
4. Johnny	11. Sammy	17. Pappy	23. Tad
5. Ronnie	12. Andy	18. Happy	24. Fred
6. Candy	13. Brandy	19. Chad	25. Jed
7. Randy			

____Oliver Twist

____Hansel & Gretel

____Goldilocks & the 3 Bears

____Macbeth

____Cinderella

____Snow White

____Sleeping Beauty

____Pinocchio

____Peter Pan

____Hamlet

____Black Beauty

____Scrooge

____Jack & the Beanstalk

____Jack & Jill

____Red Riding Hood

____Old King Cole

____Santa Claus

____Nancy Drew

____The Hardy Boys

____Moby Dick

____Humpty Dumpty

____Alice in Wonderland

____Tom Sawyer

____Huckleberry Finn

____The Wizard of Oz

25 items

WHAT DO THEY WANT TO BE?

1. Benny	8. Andy	14. Patty	20. Willie
2. Jenny	9. Randy	15. Kitty	21. Darlene
3. Denny	10. Candy	16. Betty	22. Marlene
4. Wendy	11. Tammy	17. Lilly	23. Arlene
5. Kenny	12. Sammy	18. Billy	24. Sharlene
6. Penny	13. Pammie	19. Jill	25. Harley
7. Sandy			

____pilot   ____pharmacist   ____mayor   ____director

____veterinarian   ____actor   ____secretary   ____engineer

____physician   ____actress   ____soldier   ____teacher

____nurse   ____detective   ____writer   ____stock broker

____dentist   ____dancer   ____principal   ____banker

____lawyer   ____president   ____astronaut   ____accountant

____policeman

25 items

WHAT DID THEY SMELL?

1. bug	8. pup	14. crab	20. seal
2. frog	9. skunk	15. stag	21. ant
3. slug	10. mink	16. cat	22. snail
4. hog	11. hen	17. lamb	23. mole
5. pig	12. ram	18. kid	24. colt
6. dog	13. clam	19. rat	25. bull
7. cub			

____onions	____yeast	____roses	____skunk
____bacon	____shoe polish	____shampoo	____pine tree
____gasoline	____perfume	____cologne	____coffee
____fire	____paints	____chocolate	____cake baking
____fish	____vinegar	____vitamins	____soap
____garlic	____vanilla	____lemons	____flowers
____baking bread			

25 items

IN WHAT COUNTRIES WERE THEY BORN?

1. Jenny	8. Candy	14. Hanna	20. Sammy
2. Benny	9. Randy	15. Janet	21. Tammy
3. Denny	10. Mandy	16. Janice	22. Danny
4. Kenny	11. Lana	17. Tommy	23. Jimmy
5. Penny	12. Anna	18. Donny	24. Timmy
6. Wendy	13. Donna	19. Ronnie	25. Kitty
7. Sandy			

____England   ____Greece   ____Denmark

____Poland   ____France   ____Germany

____Scotland   ____Iceland   ____Italy

____Holland   ____Greenland   ____Norway

____Ireland   ____Newfoundland   ____Belgium

____Finland   ____Switzerland   ____Turkey

____Sweden   ____Russia   ____India

____Wales   ____Austria   ____Egypt

____Spain

25 items

WHAT DID THEY DO?

1. Mr. Jones	8. Master Smith	14. Mrs. Hall	20. Master Bell
2. Mrs. Jones	9. Mr. Miller	15. Miss Hall	21. Mr. Shaw
3. Miss Jones	10. Mrs. Miller	16. Master Hall	22. Mrs. Shaw
4. Master Jones	11. Miss Miller	17. Mr. Bell	23. Miss Shaw
5. Mr. Smith	12. Master Miller	18. Mrs. Bell	24. Master Shaw
6. Mrs. Smith	13. Mr. Hall	19. Miss Bell	25. Mrs. Hill
7. Miss Smith			

____worked quickly   ____walked carefully   ____asked politely

____acted courteously   ____danced gracefully   ____dressed beautifully

____looked angrily   ____printed neatly   ____played well

____talked rapidly   ____read frequently   ____jumped happily

____answered correctly   ____sewed occasionally ____barked loudly

____drove recklessly   ____graded fairly   ____spoke clearly

____stood quietly   ____felt badly   ____sang well

____dug deeply   ____stopped suddenly   ____acted patiently

____held on tightly

25 items

DESCRIBE EACH PERSON

1. Gail	8. Paula	14. Wendy	20. Sherry
2. Belle	9. Polly	15. Benny	21. Mary
3. Jill	10. Penny	16. Donna	22. Jerry
4. Lilly	11. Denny	17. Donnie	23. Larry
5. Milly	12. Jenny	18. Robbie	24. Clara
6. Nell	13. Kenny	19. Robin	25. Sarah
7. Paul			

____kind	____friendly	____quiet	____healthy
____polite	____generous	____cheerful	____lonely
____intelligent	____wealthy	____jolly	____honest
____old	____educated	____beautiful	____cruel
____young	____careful	____sad	____poor
____clever	____successful	____religious	____rude
____lazy			

25 items

WHERE DID THE CHILDREN GO?

1. Dick	8. Gay	14. Dean	20. Phil
2. Vic	9. Kay	15. Helen	21. Will
3. Nick	10. Jay	16. Ellen	22. Gill
4. Rick	11. Eve	17. Allen	23. Belle
5. May	12. Steve	18. Jill	24. Mel
6. Fay	13. Jean	19. Bill	25. Nell
7. Ray			

_____zoo   _____ocean   _____circus   _____country

_____park   _____motel   _____party   _____wedding

_____play   _____museum   _____dance   _____restaurant

_____theater   _____castle   _____airport   _____funeral

_____school   _____farm   _____hospital   _____concert

_____church   _____beach   _____parade   _____opera

_____lake

25 items

WHAT DID THE MAILMAN BRING?

1. Bess	8. Sis	14. Rhonda	20. Winnie
2. Fess	9. Paul	15. Bonnie	21. Wendy
3. Tess	10. Paula	16. Bobbie	22. Penny
4. Wes	11. Wally	17. Donna	23. Robin
5. Gus	12. Robbie	18. Donald	24. Peter
6. Chris	13. Ronnie	19. Donnie	25. Tina
7. Les			

____magazine

____newspaper

____newsletter

____Christmas card

____valentine

____invitation

____thank-you note

____report card

____catalog

____note of sympathy

____note of congratulations

____a phone bill

____business letter

____telegram

____advertisements

____Easter card

____birthday card

____birthday present

____postcard

____bus ticket

____calendar

____license plates

____surprises

____check

____book

25 items

WHAT DID THEY WEAR?

1. Ann	8. John	14. Jenny	20. Doug
2. Dan	9. Don	15. Wendy	21. Kitty
3. Jan	10. Ron	16. Kenny	22. Chrissy
4. Nan	11. Sandy	17. Penny	23. Missy
5. Pam	12. Randy	18. Timmy	24. Sissy
6. Sam	13. Cindy	19. Jimmy	25. Sonny
7. Tom			

____glasses	____blouse	____shoes	____necklace
____hat	____sweater	____suit	____vest
____dress	____pajamas	____socks	____slacks
____coat	____shorts	____hose	____jeans
____shirt	____jacket	____watch	____hearing aid
____skirt	____boots	____bracelet	____raincoat
____pants			

25 items

WHAT PRESIDENTS DID THEY VOTE FOR?

1. Mary	8. Sherry	14. Holly	20. Bob
2. Larry	9. Sarah	15. Molly	21. Robin
3. Jerry	10. Erin	16. Dolly	22. John
4. Harry	11. Karen	17. Laura	23. Scott
5. Perry	12. Darrin	18. Olive	24. Dot
6. Terry	13. Sharon	19. Colin	25. Maude
7. Gary			

____John Adams

____John Quincy Adams

____John Kennedy

____Lyndon Johnson

____Andrew Jackson

____Thomas Jefferson

____Gerald Ford

____Harry Truman

____Teddy Roosevelt

____Franklin Roosevelt

____Abraham Lincoln

____James Polk

____Franklin Pierce

____Warren Harding

____William Taft

____Calvin Coolidge

____James Monroe

____James Madison

____Herbert Hoover

____Woodrow Wilson

____Zachary Taylor

____Dwight Eisenhower

____Andrew Johnson

____Jimmy Carter

____Ulysses Grant

25 items

WHAT CITIES DID THEY VISIT?

1. Graham	8. Anna	14. Tim	20. Lora
2. Ann	9. Hannah	15. Wynne	21. Nora
3. Lance	10. Janet	16. Lynne	22. Flora
4. Dan	11. Fran	17. Ken	23. Harold
5. Pam	12. Kim	18. Dora	24. Gerald
6. Sam	13. Jim	19. Cora	25. Carol
7. Grant			

____London	____Berlin	____Bombay	____Honolulu
____Rome	____Paris	____Bangkok	____Liverpool
____Moscow	____Oslo	____Brussels	____Bern
____Cairo	____Calcutta	____Madrid	____Hamburg
____Tokyo	____Lisbon	____Naples	____Venice
____Dublin	____Warsaw	____Athens	____Seville
____Bonn			

25 items

WHAT BODY OF WATER DID THEY CROSS?

1. Judy	8. Hugh	14. Allen	20. Linda
2. Lucy	9. Drew	15. Alvin	21. Freda
3. Rudy	10. Lou	16. Calvin	22. Greta
4. Ruby	11. Sue	17. Duke	23. Emma
5. Susie	12. Stu	18. Edna	24. Hedda
6. Trudy	13. Ralph	19. Brenda	25. Ed
7. Luke			

____Hudson Bay   ____North Sea   ____Mississippi River

____English Channel   ____Baltic Sea   ____Congo River

____Irish Sea   ____Arctic Ocean   ____Yukon River

____Japan Sea   ____Atlantic Ocean   ____Orange River

____Coral Sea   ____Pacific Ocean   ____Great Salt Lake

____Black Sea   ____Indian Ocean   ____Ohio River

____Red Sea   ____Nile River   ____Reindeer Lake

____Mediterranean Sea   ____Amazon River   ____St. Lawrence River

____Gulf of Mexico

25 items

WHAT ANIMALS DID THEY SEE AT THE ZOO?

1. Clay
2. Gray
3. Hayes
4. Ames
5. James
6. Haines
7. Daisy

8. Percy
9. Bernie
10. Ernie
11. Kirby
12. Herbie
13. Erma

14. Myrna
15. Verna
16. Bertha
17. Herman
18. Kermit
19. Eartha

20. Martha
21. Marsha
22. Mark
23. Marva
24. Shirley
25. Curley

____elephant
____zebra
____anteater
____chimpanzee
____rhinoceros
____lion
____tiger

____leopard
____Polar bear
____black bear
____panda bear
____antelope
____gorilla

____orangutan
____giraffe
____hippopotamus
____camel
____cheetah
____bison

____baboon
____kangaroo
____yak
____caribou
____dingo
____moose

25 items

WHAT DID THEY DO?

1. mother	3. sister	5. daughter	7. aunt
2. father	4. brother	6. cousin	8. uncle

____mowed   ____grated   ____splashed   ____knitted

____sewed   __ __hated   ____dashed   ____weeded

____towed   ____paced   ____mashed   ____panted

____rode   ____hopped   ____flashed   ____planted

____skated   ____chopped   ____wished   ____danced

____baked   ____shopped   ____stitched   ____pranced

____raked   ____flopped   ____fished   ____glanced

____framed   ____washed   ____finished   ____sweated

____blamed   ____talked   ____kissed   ____patted

____stated   ____knocked   ____wanted   ____prayed

____dated   ____rocked   ____thought   ____played

____braided   ____dropped   ____greeted   ____raided

____waited   ____waded

50 items

WHAT WERE THEY DOING?

1. mother   3. sister   5. daughter

2. father   4. brother   6. teacher

___teaching	___singing	___climbing	___cheating
___preaching	___blinking	___diving	___freezing
___reaching	___skipping	___driving	___sneezing
___praying	___swimming	___riding	___dreaming
___playing	___fishing	___hiding	___cleaning
___skating	___wishing	___sliding	___sleeping
___waiting	___sitting	___crying	___thinking
___painting	___knitting	___lying	___sewing
___baking	___washing	___dining	___growing
___raking	___racing	___frying	___blowing
___waking	___drinking	___flying	___rowing
___shaking	___laying	___eating	___throwing
___swinging			___winking

50 items

STORES & SHOPS

1. drugstore
2. grocery store
3. barber shop
4. florist

5. post office
6. card shop
7. dairy store
8. dress shop

9. shoe store
10. book store
11. state store
12. pet shop

13. bakery
14. toy store
15. sport shop
16. music store

____wine	____clothes	____mint	____cheese
____vine	____rose	____gun	____wreath
____lime	____oats	____rinse	____gin
____dime	____hose	____soap	____pin
____rhyme	____rice	____cone	____clove
____swine	____dice	____bone	____chest
____mum	____ice	____phone	____vest
____pie	____stein	____chintz	____desk
____plum	____mice	____rope	____mesh
____gum	____spice	____horn	____pup
____bun	____print	____corn	____pen
____rum	____tint	____cream	____boat
____drum			____ivy

50 items

WHAT WERE IN THE SCHOOLROOMS?

1. health room
2. art room
3. lunch room
4. storeroom
5. music room
6. principal's office

7. library
8. gym
9. locker room
10. sewing room
11. cooking room

12. science lab
13. language lab
14. teacher's room
15. speech room
16. shop

____teacher

____bleacher

____speaker

____basket

____cabinet

____planet

____blanket

____showers

____flowers

____needles

____beetles

____spindles

____chisels

____coffee

____toffee

____smock

____chalk

____pattern

____sweater

____pot

____pastels

____records

____leopards

____flippers

____clippers

25 items

130

WHAT WERE IN THE ROOMS?

1. kitchen	5. dining room	9. powder room
2. bedroom	6. living room	10. sewing room
3. bathroom	7. family room	11. game room
4. playroom	8. laundry room	

____pickle   ____butter   ____fryer   ____holly

____nickel   ____shutter   ____mirror   ____dresser

____fiddle   ____putter   ____quarter   ____letter

____kitten   ____funnel   ____dollar   ____bucket

____rattle   ____truffle   ____collar   ____window

____saddle   ____dryer   ____dolly   ____minnow

____mantle

25 items

WHAT DID THEY SEE ON THE PLANETS?

1. Earth   4. Mars   6. Pluto   8. Jupiter

2. Mercury   5. Saturn   7. Neptune   9. Uranus

3. Venus

____seaweeds   ____blue cakes   ____lead shells

____green trees   ____true lakes   ____cherry stars

____green cheese   ____two drakes   ____berry jars

____lean fleas   ____bent trout   ____hairy cars

____cream cheese   ____dead hounds   ____melon pies

____mean bees   ____bread mounds   ____pillow skies

____round holes   ____red cows   ____yellow flies

____brown moles   ____bear wells   ____thread clouds

____shoe snakes

25 items

WHAT 2 THINGS DID THEY HAVE FOR DINNER?

1. peas   4. peaches   6. cheese   8. beef
2. beans   5. meat   7. greens   9. leeks
3. beets   10. cream

____corn   ____ham   ____cole slaw   ____tomatoes

____chicken   ____turkey   ____spaghetti   ____crab

____carrots   ____weiners   ____pizza   ____lobster

____bread   ____soup   ____hamburgers   ____rice

____potatoes   ____lamb   ____sandwiches   ____omelet

____fish   ____salad   ____bacon   ____rolls

____steak

25 items

WHEN ARE THEIR BIRTHDAYS?

1. January	4. April	7. July	10. October
2. February	5. May	8. August	11. November
3. March	6. June	9. September	12. December

____Sherry   ____Terry   ____Jackie   ____Danny

____Mary   ____Barry   ____Betty   ____Kenny

____Larry   ____Tammy   ____Eddie   ____Jenny

____Gary   ____Sammy   ____Betsy   ____Lenny

____Harry   ____Annie   ____Katie   ____Benny

____Jerry   ____Patty   ____Debbie   ____Denny

____Perry

25 items

ANSWERS FOR SECTION 5

FILL IN THE BLANK (INITIAL CONSONANT)

b oom	**c** ake	**p** ale	**p** ave
r oom	**w** ake	**g** ale	**c** ave
d oom	**f** ake	**h** ale	**w** ave
z oom	**r** ake	**m** ale	**s** ave
l oom	**t** ake	**k** ale	**r** ave

w ool	**g** ame	**c** ane	**s** eek
c ool	**d** ame	**s** ane	**m** eek
f ool	**s** ame	**l** ane	**r** eek
t ool	**t** ame	**p** ane	**w** eek
p ool	**n** ame	**v** ane	**m** eek

b ook	**r** ace	**g** ape	**m** eat
c ook	**l** ace	**c** ape	**s** eat
l ook	**p** ace	**n** ape	**n** eat
t ook	**m** ace	**t** ape	**h** eat
h ook	**f** ace	**r** ape	**b** eat

t oot	**j** ade	**c** are	**r** eal
m oot	**w** ade	**f** are	**s** eal
b oot	**f** ade	**m** are	**m** eal
l oot	**m** ade	**r** are	**d** eal
h oot	**b** ade	**w** are	**h** eal

w ore	**w** age	**r** ate	**w** eed
s ore	**p** age	**l** ate	**s** eed
c ore	**r** age	**m** ate	**d** eed
m ore	**c** age	**h** ate	**f** eed
p ore	**s** age	**d** ate	**r** eed

100 items

FILL IN THE BLANK (INITIAL CONSONANT)

p ain	l ike	t ime	w ing
m ain	h ike	l ime	k ing
l ain	d ike	r ime	s ing
r ain	b ike	d ime	r ing
g ain	p ike	m ime	d ing
j ob	d ice	w ire	w est
s ob	r ice	f ire	j est
r ob	m ice	h ire	r est
c ob	l ice	s ire	b est
m ob	n ice	t ire	n est
f air	s ide	s ight	m oss
h air	w ide	f ight	t oss
l air	h ide	l ight	b oss
p air	r ide	n ight	l oss
m air	t ide	t ight	r oss
g old	r ind	h ive	b elt
h old	f ind	f ive	w elt
f old	k ind	l ive	f elt
t old	w ind	d ive	m elt
s old	b ind	j ive	p elt
w ine	f ile	l aid	m atch
d ine	p ile	m aid	h atch
l ine	t ile	r aid	b atch
n ine	v ile	s aid	c atch
f ine	b ile	p aid	l atch

100 items

FILL IN THE BLANK (INITIAL CONSONANT)

_c_ at	_c_ all	_y_ am	_b_ ar
_m_ at	_t_ all	_j_ am	_c_ ar
_s_ at	_m_ all	_dr_ am	_f_ ar
_r_ at	_f_ all	_t_ am	_t_ ar
_f_ at	_w_ all	_h_ am	_j_ ar

_c_ an	_m_ ail	_r_ ug	_s_ ay
_f_ an	_j_ ail	_j_ ug	_m_ ay
_m_ an	_dn_ ail	_db_ ug	_r_ ay
_r_ an	_t_ ail	_h_ ug	_w_ ay
_t_ an	_f_ ail	_d_ ug	_d_ ay

_b_ un	_w_ et	_w_ ill	_f_ og
_r_ un	_gj_ et	_f_ ill	_d_ og
_f_ un	_dm_ et	_k_ ill	_l_ og
_s_ un	_s_ et	_m_ ill	_j_ og
_g_ un		_b_ ill	_dh_ og

_f_ in	_p_ ot	_y_ ell	_l_ ip
_w_ in	_g_ ot	_b_ ell	_r_ ip
_s_ in	_dh_ ot	_f_ ell	_s_ ip
_t_ in	_j_ ot	_s_ ell	_h_ ip
_p_ in	_dn_ ot	_t_ ell	_t_ ip

_b_ ad	_w_ ig	_y_ ear	_c_ ap
_m_ ad	_p_ ig	_f_ ear	_s_ ap
_s_ ad	_j_ ig	_n_ ear	_t_ ap
_h_ ad	_df_ ig	_h_ ear	_g_ ap
_f_ ad	_b_ ig	_r_ ear	_dm_ ap

100 items

FILL IN THE BLANK (INITIAL CONSONANT OR BLEND)

sh ack	**cl** ump	**j** eep	**z** ipper
j ack	**th** ump	**sh** eep	**cl** ipper
st ack	**j** ump	**st** eep	**ch** ipper
s ack		**s** eep	
	th y		**st** ar
ch in	**sh** y	**j** aw	**j** ar
s in	**st** y	**s** aw	
th in		**th** aw	**z** one
sh in	**cl** ay		**st** one
	g ay	**s** at	**sh** one
st ew	**j** ay	**th** at	
ch ew		**ch** at	**g** ap
J ew	**st** op		**ch** ap
	ch op	**ch** unk	**s** ap
st ick	**s** op	**j** unk	**z** ap
s ick	**cl** op	**s** unk	
ch ick			**g** un
th ick	**j** am	**th** ink	**st** un
cl ick	**cl** am	**cl** ink	**s** un
	sh am	**s** ink	**sh** un
z ip			
cl ip	**ch** amp	**s** ore	**J** ill
s ip	**cl** amp	**sh** ore	**ch** ill
sh ip		**ch** ore	**st** ill
	z est	**st** ore	
sh ock	**ch** est		**s** ale
s ock	**j** est	**g** ave	**st** ale
cl ock		**s** ave	**g** ale
j ock	**j** ug	**sh** ave	
	ch ug		
th an		**sh** erry	
cl an	**g** um	**ch** erry	
J an	**ch** um	**J** erry	

100 items

FILL IN THE BLANK (INITIAL BLENDS)

_gr_ am	_ch_ in	_cr_ ate	_st_ oop
_cl_ am	_gr_ in	_st_ ate	_dr_ oop
_sl_ am	_sp_ in	_gr_ ate	_tr_ oop
_cr_ am	_th_ in		
_dr_ am		_sc_ are	_sw_ ing
_sh_ am	_fl_ ake	_sp_ are	_st_ ing
	_br_ ake	_gl_ are	_fl_ ing
_br_ an	_sn_ ake	_fl_ are	_cl_ ing
_cl_ an	_st_ ake	_sn_ are	_br_ ing
_th_ an	_dr_ ake		
_sp_ an		_tr_ ip	_sm_ ash
	_sp_ ell	_cl_ ip	_cr_ ash
_st_ and	_sw_ ell	_fl_ ip	_cl_ ash
_bl_ and	_sm_ ell	_gr_ ip	_fl_ ash
_br_ and			_tr_ ash
_gl_ and	_bl_ ed	_br_ ide	_st_ ash
	_sp_ ed	_gl_ ide	_br_ ash
_st_ ick	_sl_ ed	_sn_ ide	
_br_ ick	_br_ ed		_fl_ at
_ch_ ick	_fl_ ed	_gr_ eet	_sp_ at
_cl_ ick	_sh_ ed	_fl_ eet	_th_ at
_fl_ ick		_sl_ eet	_sl_ at
	_st_ ack	_sh_ eet	_ch_ at
_br_ im	_cr_ ack	_str_ eet	_br_ at
_gr_ im	_bl_ ack		
_tr_ im	_sm_ ack	_st_ eer	_dr_ eam
_sw_ im	_sn_ ack	_ch_ eer	_st_ eam
	_tr_ ack	_sh_ eer	_cr_ eam
_gr_ oom	_fl_ ack	_sn_ eer	_gl_ eam
_gl_ oom			
_bl_ oom			

100 items

FILL IN THE BLANK (INITIAL BLENDS)

_br_ ain	_tr_ ip	_cr_ y	_bl_ ue
_dr_ ain	_dr_ ip	_dr_ y	_tr_ ue
_st_ ain	_sh_ ip	_fl_ y	_gl_ ue
_gr_ ain	_fl_ ip	_tr_ y	
_ch_ ain	_cl_ ip	_sl_ y	_fl_ ew
		_fr_ y	_bl_ ew
			_dr_ ew
_cr_ op	_sh_ ap		_br_ ew
_st_ op	_cl_ ap	_sw_ ing	_st_ ew
_ch_ op	_fl_ ap	_st_ ing	
_dr_ op	_tr_ ap	_br_ ing	_tr_ ee
_sh_ op	_ch_ ap		_gl_ ee
		_st_ air	_fl_ ee
_st_ ag	_fl_ at	_fl_ air	
_br_ ag	_th_ at	_ch_ air	_fl_ ow
_fl_ ag	_sl_ at		_gr_ ow
_dr_ ag	_sp_ at	_br_ ave	_bl_ ow
_cr_ ag	_br_ at	_sl_ ave	_sn_ ow
		_gr_ ave	_cr_ ow
		_cr_ ave	
_cr_ ock	_st_ ay	_sh_ ave	
_cl_ ock	_cl_ ay		_bl_ ot
_st_ ock	_gr_ ay	_sp_ ill	_cl_ ot
_bl_ ock	_sl_ ay	_dr_ ill	_sp_ ot
_fl_ ock	_pr_ ay	_ch_ ill	_tr_ ot
		_fr_ ill	_sh_ ot
		_gr_ ill	
_sc_ ore	_sh_ ade		
_st_ ore	_sp_ ade	_sp_ ine	
_sn_ ore	_gr_ ade	_sh_ ine	
_sh_ ore	_bl_ ade	_br_ ine	
_sp_ ore	_tr_ ade	_th_ ine	
	_br_ oke		
	_sm_ oke		
	_ch_ oke		

FILL IN THE BLANK (FINAL CONSONANT)

pu _p_	mu _g_	ja _m_	mo _p_
pu _b_	mu _d_	ja _r_	mo _b_
pu _n_	mu _m_	ja _b_	mo _m_
pu _g_		ja _g_	mo _d_
pu _t_			
	gu _n_		
	gu _t_	ga _g_	gri _m_
to _p_	gu _m_	ga _b_	gri _p_
to _g_		ga _s_	gri _t_
to _t_		ga _d_	gri _n_
to _m_	la _g_	ga _m_	gri _d_
to _d_	la _p_		
	la _b_		
	la _x_	ru _n_	bra _g_
no _g_	la _d_	ru _b_	bra _n_
no _t_		ru _t_	bra _t_
no _b_		ru _m_	bra _d_
no _n_	do _g_	ru _g_	
	do _t_		
	do _n_		sli _m_
pa _t_		le _t_	sli _t_
pa _r_		le _d_	sli _p_
pa _d_	na _p_	le _g_	sli _d_
pa _n_	na _g_	le _k_	
pa _l_	na _b_		
	Na _n_		sla _p_
		dra _m_	sla _m_
ro _b_		dra _g_	sla _b_
ro _d_	tri _p_	dra _b_	sla _g_
ro _t_	tri _m_		sla _t_
		sta _g_	
fla _b_	gra _m_	sta _b_	cla _p_
fla _g_	gra _b_	sta _r_	cla _m_
fla _t_		sta _n_	cla _n_
fla _x_			cla _d_
fla _k_			

100 items

FILL IN THE BLANK (FINAL CONSONANT)

co _d_	ra _n_	di _g_	bu _g_
co _n_	ra _t_	di _gp_	bu _gd_
co _p_	ra _m_	di _gd_	bu _n_
co _pb_	ra _g_	di _m_	bu _t_
co _t_	ra _gp_		
		fa _n_	cu _p_
		fa _t_	cu _pb_
bi _b_	ca _b_	fa _d_	cu _d_
bi _n_	ca _n_	fa _g_	cu _t_
bi _t_	ca _p_		
bi _d_	ca _pt_		
bi _g_		ha _m_	be _g_
		ha _d_	be _gt_
	si _p_	ha _t_	be _d_
wa _x_	si _pn_	ha _s_	be _n_
wa _g_	si _t_		
wa _gr_	si _x_	li _t_	da _m_
		li _p_	da _b_
		li _pd_	da _d_
ba _g_	sa _g_		da _n_
ba _gt_	sa _gd_	ma _d_	
ba _d_	sa _t_	ma _n_	
ba _n_	sa _p_	ma _p_	fi _x_
		ma _pt_	fi _n_
		ma _m_	fi _t_
ta _gx_	ri _m_		fi _g_
ta _gx_	ri _pb_		fi _gb_
ta _n_	ri _pb_	bo _x_	
ta _p_	ri _g_	bo _g_	hi _p_
ta _pm_	ri _gd_	bo _gb_	hi _pt_
ta _b_			hi _m_
	he _m_		hi _d_
jo _b_	he _n_		hi _s_
jo _t_	he _x_		
jo _g_			

100 items

FILL IN THE BLANK (FINAL BLENDS)

ma**rk**	wa**nt**	wi**nk**	li**nt**
ma**rt**	wa**sp**	wi**lt**	li**ft**
ma**th**	wa**rm**	wi**ng**	li**nk**
ma**sk**	wa**rp**	wi**nd**	li**sp**
ma**lt**	wa**rd**	wi**tch**	li**st**
ma**st**	wa**rn**		
	wa**rt**		
mi**lk**		ri**nk**	fa**st**
mi**nt**	ba**ld**	ri**ch**	fa**rm**
mi**nk**	ba**nk**	ri**ng**	fa**ct**
mi**st**	ba**nd**	ri**sk**	fa**ng**
mi**nd**	ba**lm**	ri**ft**	
			mu**ch**
	ba**th**	be**lt**	mu**st**
a**rm**	ba**rk**	be**nd**	mu**ng**
a**rt**	ba**rn**	be**nt**	
a**rk**	ba**ng**	be**st**	si**ng**
a**sk**			si**lk**
a**rch**	la**st**	fo**rk**	si**ft**
	la**nd**	fo**rm**	si**lt**
ha**rd**	la**rk**	fo**rt**	
ha**rm**	la**rd**	fo**rd**	wo**rk**
ha**rk**		fo**ld**	wo**rm**
ha**nd**			wo**rd**
ha**lt**	bo**th**	co**rn**	wo**rn**
ha**th**	bo**ld**	co**rd**	wo**n't**
	bo**lt**	co**rk**	
sa**sh**	bo**rn**	co**ld**	we**nt**
sa**nd**	bo**nd**	co**lt**	we**st**
sa**nk**		co**st**	we**ld**
sa**ng**			
sa**lt**			

100 items

FILL IN THE BLANK (SHORT VOWEL)

m_i_st	m_e_sh	j_i_g	t_e_n
m_u_st	m_a_sh	j_o_g	t_i_n
m_a_st	m_u_sh	j_u_g	t_a_n
		j_a_g	
sl_i_p	l_i_mp		h_u_tch
sl_a_p	l_a_mp	r_i_m	h_a_tch
sl_o_p	l_u_mp	r_u_m	h_i_tch
		r_a_m	
fl_o_p	t_i_ck		r_u_st
fl_i_p	t_o_ck	r_i_b	r_e_st
fl_a_p	t_u_ck	r_o_b	
	t_a_ck	r_u_b	st_i_ck
			st_o_ck
ch_o_p			st_u_ck
ch_i_p	l_a_st	r_u_g	st_a_ck
ch_a_p	l_i_st	r_i_g	
	l_u_st	r_a_g	
	l_e_st		b_a_nd
sl_i_m	l_o_st		b_e_nd
sl_u_m		r_u_mp	b_o_nd
sl_a_m		r_a_mp	
	r_u_ng	r_o_mp	
	r_a_ng		
tr_i_ck	r_i_ng		f_i_t
tr_a_ck		s_i_t	f_a_t
tr_u_ck		s_a_t	
	_i_n	s_e_t	
	_o_n		v_e_t
w_i_g	_a_n		v_a_t
w_a_g		t_o_g	
		t_a_g	
	p_a_nt	t_u_g	_e_nd
s_i_ng	p_u_nt		_a_nd
s_a_ng	p_e_nt		
s_o_ng		l_o_g	
s_u_ng		l_u_g	sp_i_n
	p_a_st	l_e_g	sp_a_n
	p_e_st	l_a_g	sp_u_n

100 items

FILL IN THE BLANK (SHORT VOWEL)

b _e_ g	m _o_ ss	p _e_ t	p _e_ p
b _a_ g	m _e_ ss	p _a_ t	p _a_ p
b _o_ g	m _a_ ss	p _o_ t	p _o_ p
b _u_ g	m _i_ ss	p _u_ t	p _u_ p
b _i_ g	m _u_ ss	p _i_ t	
			l _i_ t
g _e_ t	d _e_ ll	f _a_ n	l _e_ t
g _u_ t	d _o_ ll	f _i_ n	l _o_ t
g _o_ t	d _u_ ll	f _u_ n	
	d _i_ ll		l _u_ ck
t _o_ p		h _e_ m	l _a_ ck
t _i_ p	f _a_ ll	h _u_ m	l _i_ ck
t _a_ p	f _e_ ll	h _i_ m	l _o_ ck
	f _u_ ll	h _a_ m	
	f _i_ ll		d _u_ ck
c _a_ p		l _a_ d	d _e_ ck
c _u_ p	b _e_ ll	l _i_ d	d _i_ ck
c _o_ p	b _u_ ll	l _e_ d	d _o_ ck
	b _o_ ll		
p _a_ ck	b _i_ ll	p _u_ n	l _a_ st
p _e_ ck		p _e_ n	l _e_ st
p _i_ ck	b _e_ t	p _a_ n	l _u_ st
p _u_ ck	b _u_ t	p _i_ n	l _i_ st
	b _i_ t		l _o_ st
n _u_ t	b _a_ t	l _e_ ss	
n _e_ t		l _o_ ss	h _a_ t
n _o_ t		l _a_ ss	h _i_ t
	r _o_ d		h _u_ t
h _a_ t	r _e_ d	d _u_ g	h _o_ t
h _i_ t	r _i_ d	d _o_ g	
h _o_ t		d _i_ g	s _i_ ck
h _u_ t			s _o_ ck
			s _u_ ck
s _i_ x			s _a_ ck
s _e_ x			

100 items

b_i_ke	l_a_ce	t_i_me	l_u_te
b_a_ke	l_i_ce	t_a_me	l_a_te
w_a_de	s_o_le	t_u_ne	r_i_pe
w_i_de	s_a_le	t_i_ne	r_o_pe
		t_o_ne	r_a_pe
d_i_ve	c_a_ne		
d_o_ve	c_o_ne	f_a_me	tr_u_ce
		f_u_me	tr_a_ce
r_a_te	c_o_pe	f_i_ne	
r_i_te	c_a_pe		br_o_ke
r_o_te		d_i_me	br_a_ke
	m_o_le	d_o_me	
c_u_te	m_u_le	d_a_me	wr_o_te
k_i_te	m_a_le		wr_i_te
	m_i_le	d_i_ne	
p_a_ne		d_u_ne	fl_u_ke
p_o_ne	h_o_le		fl_a_ke
p_i_ne	h_a_le	b_o_ne	
		b_a_ne	sp_i_ce
m_i_te	w_e_'ve		sp_a_ce
m_a_te	w_o_ve	l_i_me	
m_u_te	w_a_ve	l_a_me	gr_i_pe
m_e_te	w_i_ves		gr_o_pe
		l_a_ne	gr_a_pe
_u_se	wh_a_le	l_o_ne	
_i_ce	wh_i_le	l_i_ne	sh_i_ne
_a_ce			sh_o_ne
	l_i_ke	r_o_se	
m_a_ce	l_a_ke	r_i_se	sp_o_ke
m_i_ce			sp_i_ke
	w_i_ne	r_a_ce	
c_a_ke	w_a_ne	r_i_ce	ph_a_se
c_o_ke			ph_o_ne
r_o_de			
r_i_de			
r_u_de			

100 items